Lies! Lies!! Lies!!!

The Psychology of Deceit

Lies! Lies!! Lies!!!

The Psychology of Deceit

Charles V. Ford, M.D.

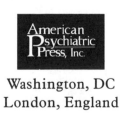

Washington, DC
London, England

Note: The author has worked to ensure that all information in this book concerning drug dosages, schedules, and routes of administration is accurate as of the time of publication and consistent with standards set by the U.S. Food and Drug Administration and the general medical community. As medical research and practice advance, however, therapeutic standards may change. For this reason and because human and mechanical errors sometimes occur, we recommend that readers follow the advice of a physician who is directly involved in their care or the care of a member of their family.

Books published by the American Psychiatric Press, Inc., represent the views and opinions of the individual authors and do not necessarily represent the policies and opinions of the Press or the American Psychiatric Association.

The essential psychological issues in each case in this book reflect real-life events. Details have been changed to ensure confidentiality. Any resemblance to actual persons, events, or locales is entirely unintentional, with the exception of names and descriptions provided in the media and cited as such.

Copyright © 1996 Charles V. Ford, M.D.
ALL RIGHTS RESERVED
Manufactured in the United States of America on acid-free paper
99 98 97 96   4 3 2 1
First Edition

American Psychiatric Press, Inc.
1400 K Street, N.W., Washington, DC   20005

Library of Congress Cataloging-in-Publication Data
Ford, Charles V., 1937–
    Lies!, lies!, lies! : the psychology of deceit / Charles V. Ford.
      p.   cm.
    Includes bibliographical references and index.
    ISBN 0-88048-739-9
    1. Deception.   2. Self-deception.   3. Truthfulness and falsehood.
I. Title.
BF637.D42F67   1995
153.8'3—dc20   95-25312
                                           CIP

British Library Cataloguing in Publication Data
A CIP record is available from the British Library.

This book is for my children:
Chuck, Scott, Katherine, John, Marc.

May they successfully navigate the
troubled seas of truth and deceit.

Contents

Acknowledgments

A number of persons have made substantial contributions to the formulation and preparation of this book. Marc Hollender, M.D., and Bryan King, M.D., were collaborators in previously published work. Virginia Abernethy, Ph.D., Russell Gardner, Jr., M.D., Jack G. Modell, M.D., and Loren Pancratz, Ph.D., reviewed portions of this manuscript and provided provocative and innovative ideas, useful suggestions, and reference materials. Other persons with whom I have discussed ideas in the book and who have made intellectual contributions include Roy N. Aruffo, M.D., Douglas Drossman, M.D., Arthur M. Freeman III, M.D., Thomas R. Garrick, M.D., Frederick G. Guggenheim, M.D., Lisa Gonzenbach, L.C.S.W., José L. Ochoa, M.D., Ph.D., Graeme Smith, M.D., Herman Willcutt, Ph.D., and the late Robert Kellner, M.D., Ph.D. I appreciate the fine work of the editorial staff of the American Psychiatric Press, particularly the careful attention and skilled editing of the manuscript by Alisa Guerzon, Project Editor, and the enthusiasm and support for the book, since its infancy, from Claire Reinburg, Editorial Director.

Preface

My scientific interest in deception began with my contact with psychiatric and medical patients who, as compulsive liars, told fantastic yet somehow believable stories in an effort to make themselves more interesting. Later, I became increasingly aware of the almost constant barrage of lies that one experiences in day-to-day life—from children, politicians, salespeople, advertisers, colleagues, friends, relatives, and even oneself.

Lying is a ubiquitous yet, from a psychological perspective, understudied phenomenon. Why lying should be the subject of so little scrutiny is of interest in itself. Perhaps it is because lying is such an intensely emotional issue. Adults tell children that there is nothing worse than a liar. In the age of chivalry, calling someone a liar was grounds for a challenge to a duel. Despite such attitudes about the evils of lying, we are all liars: we lie to others, and we lie to ourselves. If lying is so prevalent, why is it regarded as so bad, and why has it been the subject of so little study?

Noting the scarce psychiatric information available about the subject of prevarication, my colleagues Drs. Bryan King and Marc Hollender and I reviewed the medical literature on lying and wrote a review article that was published in 1988 in the *American Journal of Psychiatry.* We attempted to be objective in our approach rather than to take a moral position. The response to this article was fascinating. Several newspapers, including the *New York Times* and the *Boston Globe,* published feature articles based on our work, particularly emphasizing our ideas about the role of personality in lying. One newspaper columnist, without mentioning us specifically by name, expressed the opinion that society was in trouble because by not taking a moral stance (condemning lying), we (psychiatrists) were in essence condoning it.

As a result of this publicity, my colleagues and I were interviewed on a number of television and radio programs, including some that permitted listeners or viewers to call in with questions. This media exposure provided us and the general public with new information about lying. It was personally gratifying to receive letters from all parts of the United States. Some persons confessed that they were compulsive liars and wrote that they agreed with our proposed formulations as to why they lied. Family members of liars wrote to say that they were helped by what they had learned about compulsive lying, particularly the neurological substrates of this disorder. They told us the information helped them become more understanding of their relative.

Many of the questions directed to me about lying related to one or more of the following areas: How can you tell when someone is lying? Do lie detectors work? Should one be "truthful" about extramarital affairs? Is it always wrong to tell a lie? Why do politicians tell so many lies? What do you do when you know that your child is lying? Of course, questions that deal primarily with issues of morality are not easily answered by a scientific approach. Others, such as how lie detectors work and their degree of accuracy, are more subject to an objective description.

My intention in writing this book is to provide up-to-date information on these popular interests. I hope to go beyond that goal and stimulate interest in the concept that lying is part of the interface between a person's internal and external worlds. By this last statement, I suggest that there is an internal world composed of beliefs, fantasies, and perceived realities, and there is an external world of shared beliefs, or "reality." At the interface between these two "worlds," we lie if we deceive others as to what we believe in our personal internal world, or we engage in self-deception if we distort or change information as it passes from the external world into the internal world. In psychoanalytic terms, the function that controls this interface is called the *ego*. I conclude that lying, self-deception, and the assessment of reality are closely related to one another.

The reader of this book who expects to learn how to better detect the lies of others will learn that it is difficult to do so and that it may not, in fact, be in one's best interests to do so. Furthermore, it may not be desirable to learn how to lie more skillfully. Questions about morality and lying are to a large extent unanswerable. I hope that the reader learns to look at lying and truth-telling in a new light and learns how pervasively lies and self-deception influence human relationships and political decisions. Perhaps the most important lesson for any reader is how we use lies to deceive ourselves.

Chapter 1

Everybody Lies

Lord, Lord, how this world is given to lying.

—Shakespeare, *Henry IV, Part 1*

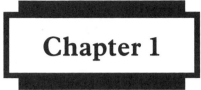

*None of us could live with a habitual truth teller;
but, thank goodness, none of us has to.*

—Mark Twain

"Lies! Lies!! Lies!!! That's all I ever hear from you! You lie when the truth would serve you better!" Rick screamed at Cindy. He had just returned from retrieving a sweater from Cindy's car, where he had found several videotapes on the front seat that she had told him she had returned days earlier. Rick became enraged. This type of lie from Cindy seemed habitual, but Rick's furious outbursts had no effect on her behavior.

Later that night, after Rick had cooled down somewhat, Cindy initiated some passionate lovemaking: "Oh, Rick, you are so sexy, so masculine, SO BIG! Oh God, how you turn me on!" Rick once again forgave Cindy's misdemeanor.

"There is nothing worse than a liar. You simply *must* tell the truth!" Ten-year-old Tyler listened to the same lecture from his mother for the umpteenth time. He had pleaded ignorance when asked how a vase was broken, but his younger sister had told his mother that it happened when Tyler threw a ball at her.

Later that afternoon, when Tyler answered a telephone call

from the pastor of the family's church, Tyler's mother said in a soft voice, "Tell him I'm not here. All he wants is a contribution for the new steeple."

"What do you mean you haven't attended classes all semester? What have we raised, a bum?" Spencer's parents were livid. They had just learned that although Spencer had registered for school at a prestigious southern university and tuition had been paid, as far as anyone could determine, Spencer had not attended a single class after the first week of school. During many phone calls, Spencer had described examinations and term papers and had even complained about his professors. In retrospect, Spencer's parents realized these conversations were fabrications. As a result of Spencer's glowing reports, they expected that their son would have a B+ or A– average for his first semester in college.

"We just don't understand it," they said to the assistant dean for student affairs. "We always had such high expectations for Spencer, and he has always pleased us."

The speaker, dressed in a blue NASA jumpsuit that reflected a rank of U.S. Marine Corps captain, enthralled the audience with the description of his flight into space aboard the shuttle *Atlantis*. He passed around an official NASA helmet for their admiring examination and then spoke of the excitement of being catapulted off an aircraft carrier in an F-18 jet fighter and going in "fast and low" to bomb Libya.

An American hero? Not quite. Not only was Robert J. Hunt not an astronaut, but he wasn't even a Marine. In fact, he didn't have a pilot's license or, according to police, even a driver's license. This impostor not only had perpetrated a successful hoax on the Experimental Aircraft Association of Boston but also had conned a young professional woman into marriage and out of thousands of dollars (Neill 1989).

Surprised and hurt by the criticism surrounding his plans to lay a wreath at the Bittburg Cemetery in West Germany, the president of the United States professed his concern about Jewish victims of Nazi Germany. He described his intense emotional reaction to what he had personally witnessed as an American army officer assisting in the liberation of a German concentration camp.

This lapse in "truth-telling" might be described as *pseudologia fantastica* (a matrix of fact and fiction, described in Chapters 2 and 7), because it was well known that Ronald Reagan never left the United States during World War II; he was a special "liaison officer" who served in Hollywood (Schaller 1992). Reagan's later disclosure that he had received a diagnosis of Alzheimer's disease may cast light on some of his statements. Pseudologia fantastica is frequently associated with cerebral dysfunction (see Chapter 3).

Paradoxes of Lying

The above illustrations demonstrate some of the many paradoxes that characterize the phenomenon of lying. Rick is furious with Cindy when he doesn't want her to lie, yet he is all too ready to hear her lies (flattery) about his sexual prowess. Tyler's mother tells him "there is nothing worse than a liar," yet a few minutes later she instructs him to lie to their minister. Spencer's parents are furious at him for lying to them, yet he is only telling them what he thinks they want to hear. If Robert Hunt, obviously a bright and talented man, had spent as much energy applying himself to genuine accomplishment as he had to masquerading as a pilot, he could probably have been a most successful man. Finally, the president of the United States lives in a fishbowl; logically, there could be no question that Ronald Reagan's fabrication would become known and that negative consequences would result.

Despite being condemned by phrases such as the one used by Tyler's mother, lies are a ubiquitous phenomenon. Much of our psychic energy is spent sorting out the day-to-day, hour-to-hour information that bombards us. "Did he really work late last night?" "Can I believe the advertisement, or is it a bait and switch?" "Has the car been as trouble-free as the seller claims?" Everyone continuously shares and receives information and must simultaneously evaluate both the effect of the information transmitted and the accuracy of information received. Only the foolish and the naive accept as true everything that is said or written. To quote a cynical old saying, "Believe nothing that you hear and only half of what you see."

Many people look back in time and see a decline in honesty and truth during the past several decades. Although this opinion is certainly debatable, no less an authority than Benjamin Bradlee, editor of *The Washington Post*, has publicly stated that lying has increased "enormously" during his lifetime (Williams 1988). Whether Bradlee is correct, or whether we are just much more aware of lying today, there is no doubt that our society is permeated with deceit.

Everybody Lies

A book based on a poll of Americans, *The Day America Told the Truth* (Patterson and Kim 1991), claimed that 90% of the people polled admitted that they were deceitful. Lies told, in order of frequency with which they were acknowledged, included lying about one's true feelings, income, accomplishments, sex life, and age.

Furthermore, many (possibly most) Americans believe that people are more dishonest now than a decade ago. In a 1987 poll by *U.S. News and World Report*–Cable News Network, 54% of the respondents thought that people were more dishonest than they were 10 years previously, and 71% indicated that they were dissatisfied with current standards of honesty (McLoughlin et al. 1987). One in four respondents thought that the president of the United States and leaders of Congress often do not tell the truth. Despite (or perhaps because of) this pervasive perception of deceit, 94% of the persons polled believed that honesty in a friend was an extremely important quality—vastly more important than any other attribute.

As an introduction to the prevalence and importance of deceit in everyday life, including in those we trust, it is useful to explore the phenomenon of lying in several different situations.

Lies for Purposes of Sexual Gratification

When it involves sexual information, accepting a lie as the truth can lead to disease or death in this age of sexually transmitted diseases. Yet, a study of dishonesty in the dating of college students found that 60% of the women stated that they had been lied to for the purposes of obtaining sex, and 34% of the men admitted to having lied for that reason. Furthermore, 4% of the men and 42% of the women stated that they would understate to a new sexual partner the number of previous partners they had had (Cochran and Mays 1990).

Dr. David Knox and his colleagues at East Carolina University investigated lies told by college students to a current or potential sexual partner (Knox et al. 1993). Ninety-two percent of the students (anonymously) reported that they had lied; the authors questioned whether the other 8% were lying about not lying. The most frequent lies of both sexes related to the correct number of previous sexual partners. Women were more likely to lie about having been sexually gratified, and men were slightly more likely to have falsely proclaimed, "I love you." The authors noted that the lies served at times to increase the chances of sexual consent but that many of the lies were to spare the feelings of the current partner. In either situation, the lies decreased potentially useful communication.

In her report on adultery, Annette Lawson (1988) estimated that about two-thirds to three-quarters of American and British married persons have extramarital affairs at some point. Of note, it may be the lying associated with infidelity rather than the sexual behavior itself that causes the most pain within the marriage. Lawson commented that in "open marriages," it is the failure to tell the other partner about an affair that constitutes unfaithfulness. She also observed that telling the spouse about an affair is often an expression of self-centeredness and hostility rather than an effort to improve communication and resolve problems. She described one woman who "confessed" her affair to appease her conscience but who had every intention of secretly continuing the extramarital liaison.

Lies in the Workplace

A recent survey by Thorndike Deland Associates estimated that one in three people "varnish the truth" or engage in out-and-out lying when seeking employment (Underwood 1993). Candidates for executive jobs are just as likely to lie as those seeking lower-level positions. The type of lie varies from falsely claiming college degrees to stretching periods of employment to cover periods of unemployment. A typical fabrication told by a man is that he played on his college football team. A typical lie told by a woman is that she was president of her sorority. Ed Andler, author of *Winning the Hiring Game* (as reported in Underwood 1993), stated that this type of lying has about doubled since the mid-1970s. One reason for the increased rate of deceit is the low risk of detection. Because employers fear lawsuits, they are reluctant to provide negative information about former employees. According to one employment service manager, most employers will now give out little more than the worker's "name, rank, and serial number" (Underwood 1993).

Lies do not stop when an applicant is hired and becomes an employee. Lies among employees of corporations are common and are motivated by a variety of reasons, including protecting one's "turf" and attempting to resolve problems, such as those encountered when reporting to two supervisors who make conflicting demands (Grover 1993a).

Lies in the workplace are not limited to employees. Jackall (1980) studied managerial style at a large bank and found that the "effective manager" had developed a number of strategies, some deceptive, to keep workers productive. The deceptive strategies included lying to workers about opportunities for advancement, deceiving overworked employees about possible forthcoming relief, displaying bursts of staged anger, playing workers off against each other by the use of innuendo, and using worker informants to gather information about their co-workers.

When an adversarial relationship develops between workers and managers, deceit becomes a frequently used tactic in the conflict. The resultant decrease in truthfulness will adversely affect the ability of the organization to fulfill its mission (Culbert and McDonough 1992).

A recent wave of restructuring (downsizing) has occurred among corporations and other organizations. Employees—including many who have worked for the same company for decades—have been laid off. Tension is high in the workplace, and many employees have experienced a loss of trust and loyalty in companies that they previously identified as "family."

Competition among co-workers for the remaining positions leads to increased fear and a lack of willingness to cooperate with one another. These conditions are counterproductive to creating a climate of trust, honest communication, and greater efficiency. Ultimately, the negative effects on the company's bottom line caused by decreased efficiency resulting from loss of morale may outweigh the savings brought by a reduced payroll.

The Lies of Advertisers

An article in one of the United States' leading advertising periodicals started with this sentence: "In 1991, truth in marketing has become as contradictory a concept as nutritional desserts." This article by Fara Warner (1991, p. 4) further stated that instead of supporting the honest attributes of their products, many advertisers "fall into a Pinocchio complex of unsubstantiated, irrelevant, or utterly false claims." This phenomenon of misleading advertising is so pronounced that one manufacturer used a deliberately exaggerated liar—"Joe Isuzu"—to create interest in its product (Lippert 1987, p. 58).

Newsweek magazine attributes to philosopher Christina Hoff Sommers the contention that television advertising is the main villain in creating a continuous barrage of "disinformation." *U.S. News and World Report* also quotes advertising executive Jerry Della Femina (whose firm was responsible for the very effective "Joe Isuzu" advertisements) as saying, "We're conceived, born, and deceived. By the time someone reaches the age of 10, he's pretty cynical" (McLoughlin et al. 1987, p. 59).

Few people would argue about the necessity of advertisements. In a large metropolitan society, advertising is the tool that producers use to communicate information to potential consumers. Conversely, consumers in need of a product search advertisements for information. Despite the usefulness of this medium of communication, few advertisers limit their advertising to providing basic information. Advertisers promote their wares by use of blatant misrepresentation, exaggeration, bait-and-switch techniques, and the subtle implication that something positive will accrue to the consumer who uses the product. I briefly discuss each of these strategies.

Blatant misrepresentation. Unfortunately, even in this relatively sophisticated society, blatant misrepresentation and bold-faced lies are not uncommon. For example, Mark Hulbert (1991), author of the *Hulbert Guide to Financial Newsletters*, found it necessary to publicly rebuke the advertising claims for Jay Schabacker's *Mutual Funds Investing* newsletter. Schabacker had claimed that Hulbert had rated his newsletter number 1, while in fact it ranked near the bottom (number 12 of 14) of Hulbert's list. One must keep in mind that the targets of Schabacker's dishonest advertisement were people with money to invest—people who are presumably not naive about financial matters.

Other advertisements with blatant misrepresentations are those that often appeal to less sophisticated consumer groups. Such advertisements may be found in certain tabloids and promise that their products will increase the size of one's penis or breasts, restore virility, or provide rapid weight loss without effort.

Exaggeration.   Advertising frequently exaggerates the attributes of a product. I remember a cartoon from decades ago featuring a street that had three hamburger stands. The first had a sign saying "best hamburgers in America," the second had a sign saying "best hamburgers in the world," but the third modestly claimed "best hamburgers on this block." Superlatives abound in advertising, and this form of advertising is more difficult to discredit than blatant lies. Such advertisements may be accompanied by a small-print disclaimer that results were obtained by "professionals" or the equivalent.

The exaggeration of a product's virtues is known as *puffery*. This advertising technique is widely used, sometimes blatantly and sometimes subtly. Puffery suggests the superiority of the advertised product through implication rather than by literal claims—"Nothing beats a great pair of L'Eggs," for example. The Federal Trade Commission (FTC) has been relatively lax in policing puffery claims, particularly those that "puff" by implication, because of the assumption that people expect advertisements to exaggerate, and therefore, astute consumers discount them (Preston 1977). However, research indicates that puffery claims are effective and influence consumers (Oliver 1979; Rotfeld and Rotzoll 1980; Wyckham 1987). Furthermore, the consumer tends to keep believing the claims of puffery after purchasing the product, even if the claims are unjustified (Oliver 1979). People need to believe that they made the right choice in buying a product, so they deceive themselves into believing that the product is superior!

Bait-and-switch techniques. *Bait and switch* is a common advertising gimmick. One well-known national retailer has been publicly censured for using this practice to bring potential consumers into its stores. There are two basic variations of bait and switch. An advertisement may offer a product (e.g., a vacuum cleaner) at a certain price. When potential buyers arrive at the store, they may be told 1) that the advertised price was for a "stripped-down" model and that for a few more dollars, a much higher quality product is available, or 2) that the advertised product has been sold out, but other models (at a higher price) are still available. The bait-and-switch technique in marketing is so prevalent that it is doubtful that any American consumer has escaped an encounter with it at least once.

Subtle implication. One of the most insidious forms of advertising is that which subtly implies that possession or use of the product will bestow certain desired characteristics on the purchaser. For example, the upscale consumer is told that purchase of a certain make of automobile will tell the world that one has "arrived," whereas advertisements for ocean cruises imply romance.

Implications (including deceptive messages) about products are frequently delivered through nonverbal communication (P. J. DePaulo 1988; Edell 1988; Stewart et al. 1987). Interestingly, but not surprisingly, these nonverbal cues are often more effective than just words because they evoke more associative thoughts and fantasies than words alone. Among the nonverbal messages found in advertisements are pictures and music. Mitchel and Olson (1981) found that constructing a visual advertisement of a kitten next to a box of facial tissue was more effective in communicating a message of "softness" than were words that described the facial tissue as soft. Music can also be used to manipulate associated ideas and moods (Stout and Leckenby 1988). For example, music can be used to associate happy social occasions with the consumption of a certain brand of beer. Deceptive advertising, by using nonverbal messages to create false implications, can be remarkably effective. Cigarette advertising provides an interesting example of nonverbal message techniques.

Cigarette advertising is remarkably sophisticated and insidiously deceitful in its appeal to the psychological vulnerabilities of children and adolescents. It has been demonstrated that RJR Nabisco's advertising campaign, which features the cartoon figure Old Joe, has been very successful among young people. "The smooth character" of Old Joe effectively appeals to an age group that is typified by awkwardness, interpersonal sensitivity, and social ineptness (DiFranza et al. 1991). In one survey, more than 90% of children recognized the Old Joe Camel cigarette logo and correctly identified it as representing a cigarette product; virtually the same percentage of the same children recognized Mickey Mouse as the logo for the Disney Channel (Fischer et al. 1991). Other cigarette advertisements imply that smoking a particular brand of cigarettes will confer sexual appeal on the smoker.

A recent article by Ballin and Johnson (1993) summarized the tactics the tobacco industry uses in its efforts to deceive the American public about the true risks of cigarette smoking. Despite overwhelming evidence, the tobacco industry continues to deny that cigarette smoking is injurious to health.

Devious advertisements that use techniques of subtle implication are not aimed solely at the poorly educated. Products such as certain types of automobiles or watches imply exclusivity and high social status via ownership of them. Advertisements and accompanying pictures for prescription drugs imply health, vigor, improved interpersonal relationships, and a more youthful appearance for patients who receive prescriptions for certain medications. Is it any wonder that physicians prescribe medications for themselves?

The above type of subtle advertising is not only very effective, but also, because of the lack of overt promises, almost impossible to regulate. One is bombarded daily with stimuli that imply that happiness can be obtained through the simple purchase and use of a product such as toothpaste.

The Lies of Politicians

Among professions, politics may have the most tarnished reputation for truth-telling. One often hears statements such as "You can't get elected if you tell the truth," or "He is always talking out of both sides of his mouth." Some people are concerned that deceit by politicians may actually be increasing and that the moral standards of our leaders may be reaching new lows (McLoughlin et al. 1987).

Although it is by no means certain that politicians lie more frequently than other people, there can be little doubt that politicians do deceive. Perhaps because of their high visibility and the fact that their actions are recorded by the media, they are caught in the act more frequently and thus appear to lie more frequently than do other persons.

The lies of a politician can be categorized as follows: 1) lies to gain election or ensure reelection (e.g., "No new taxes!"); 2) lies to pursue political policies (e.g., the fiction of an attack on United States ships in the Tonkin Gulf to justify increased bombing of North Vietnam); 3) lies to protect national security and military operations (e.g., the denial by Jimmy Carter—"I will not lie to you"—that there was a plan to attempt rescue operations for American hostages in Iran); and 4) foolish lies. Although moralists may question their justification, the first three categories appear straightforward in their motivation and implementation. But what about foolish lies? Why do politicians make false statements that are ultimately certain to do them more harm than good?

Some foolish lies have received considerable national publicity. Among them is the statement by Ronald Reagan that he personally witnessed the liberation of a German concentration camp. An obviously bright and talented man, Joseph Biden, the U.S. Senator from Delaware, not only unnecessarily plagiarized speeches from other world figures but also misrepresented his educational background ("Gary Hart and Joe Biden" 1987). Gary Hart lied about his extramarital activity and then dared the press to prove him wrong! Interestingly and inexplicably, he had also lied about his age (Dionne 1987). Ross Perot told a national ABC News audience, "I don't dig into people's personal lives. I never have," despite extensive evidence to the contrary (Alter 1992). To explain such lapses in truth-telling, one must search for psychological explanations rather than political motives (see Chapters 5 and 13).

The Lies of Physicians and Their Patients

A study reported in the *Journal of the American Medical Association* investigated hypothetical circumstances under which a physician would deceive a patient or a patient's family (Novack et al. 1989). Seventy percent of the physicians who responded to a questionnaire indicated that they would deceive an insurance company in order to obtain payment for a diagnostic or screening test (such as a mammogram) for a woman of limited financial means. In order to save a marriage, a majority of physicians would participate in a plan to deceive the wife of a man who had contracted gonorrhea in an extramarital affair. In fact, 87% of the physicians indicated that deception to patients is justified under some circumstances. Usually such circumstances are those that would clearly benefit the patient. However, physicians may be more honest in the abstract than in practice and may, self-servingly, see themselves in a favorable light. It is important to note that the physicians in this research study saw themselves as infrequently deceptive but judged other physicians to be more deceptive than themselves.

In the past two to three decades, physicians have been enjoined to be more honest with patients about both diagnosis and prognosis, to provide detailed information, and to obtain consent for diagnostic or therapeutic procedures (Novack et al. 1979). Although there have unquestionably been changes in their behavior and physicians are now more candid than they previously were, there also can be little question that physicians conceal or slant unfavorable news. Patients often receive more details about favorable outcomes than about negative results. Physicians offer the dying cancer patient hope with statements such as "Research is developing new and effective treatments every day." It is also well established that patients hear the information that they wish to hear and exclude the remainder from their consciousness (G. Robinson and Merav 1976).

Interestingly, a new issue being discussed is whether doctors are *too truthful* to their patients and whether there is any value in such "terminal candor"; European physicians have criticized their American counterparts as being too brutal (Lear 1993). Truthfulness in medicine also raises fascinating ethical dilemmas. Should one always tell the complete truth to a patient, when it has been established that hope and optimism (even when unjustified) will decrease the likelihood of dying during or after an operation and will, in fact, extend life (Kennedy and Bakst 1966)?

When doctors lie, is it only out of altruism, or are other factors at play? Deceit, as seen in several examples, may be self-serving. Physicians may lie to deny or displace their culpability for poor outcomes among ill patients. They may also lie to deny their ignorance or powerlessness to heal certain diseases. Deception may help a physician to avoid the interpersonal discomfort and intrapsychic conflict of talking openly about disability or death. Physicians, as a group, may not be particularly honest. Intense competitive pressures in the field of medicine often lead students to cheat in college, medical school, and residency training (Petersdorf 1989).

A recent study at one medical school, which surveyed both students and faculty, yielded the opinion that approximately 10% of students cheated on examinations (R. E. Anderson and Obenshain 1994). The authors of this study stated that cheating among students may be increasing. Furthermore, the authors believed cheating was no more frequent at their medical school than at others.

Every winter, graduating medical school seniors participate in a national "match" day that announces which residency training program has accepted them. There is a great deal of competition; residency programs want the best students, and students want to train at the most prestigious hospitals. This annual "mating game" has achieved such a reputation for deceit that neither party is advised to take the statements of the other party at face value (Boudreaux 1992). The most common form of deceit (on the part of both parties) is to indicate greater interest than is actually held, in the hope of increasing the other party's interest. For example, a senior student may tell a training program that it is his or her first choice, when in fact it may be his or her third or fourth choice.

Medical school faculty often are not paragons of virtue themselves. Because of career pressures, some faculty members have turned to research fraud. Medical ethics is usually of low priority to both faculty and students, and the topic is poorly taught in medical school. Students may regard telling overt lies as unethical but may not realize that telling half-truths or failing to correct misperceptions is equally deceptive and, thus, equally unethical.

People may be quick to blame doctors for their lack of honesty, but patients are also deceptive (Pancratz 1989). Squire and colleagues (1991) found that 14% of patients with allergic asthma who were smokers (a significant risk factor for severe complications of asthma) had concealed this information from their physicians. Patients (or people applying to the military, for employment, or for insurance coverage) may conceal risk factors for human immunodeficiency virus (HIV) or substance abuse (Dunbar and Rehm 1992; Potterat et al. 1987).

In a study reported in the *Journal of the American Medical Association* (Blumberg et al. 1971), it was found that, unknown to their physicians, at least 60% of young psychiatrically hospitalized patients were covertly using drugs of abuse. Testing for these drugs was accomplished under the guise of collecting urine for a survey of urinary creatinine, a measure of kidney function. However, as cogently observed by Szasz (1972), not only the patients were deceptive but also the doctors who had deceived the patients as to the nature of the test.

Dr. Latkin and colleagues (1993) from Johns Hopkins University in Baltimore found that men who were at high risk for contracting HIV infection (e.g., drug users who shared intravenous drug needles or recipients of anal intercourse) were often self-deceptive and denied these behaviors to their physicians.

The practice of obtaining controlled substances from unsuspecting (or passively acquiescent) physicians and pharmacists is widespread. Addicts learn that lying to physicians is just as effective, and has considerably less risk, than committing crimes such as burglary to obtain drugs (Goldman 1987a, 1987b, 1987c).

Some people make a career of producing or feigning a disease (e.g., a nondiabetic person injecting himself or herself with insulin) and conceal this vital information from their physicians. These "professional patients" are described in Chapter 8.

The Lies of Scientists

If there is any one area of human endeavor in which deceit should be unexpected, it is in science. By definition, scientists seek knowledge (truth), and the scientific method requires rigorous investigation, including efforts to seek alternative explanations for one's findings, in order to explore new areas of knowledge.

Two books (Broad and Wade 1982; D. J. Miller and Hersen 1992) document that scientists may also have significant lapses in their truth-seeking behavior, engaging in various forms of deceit and fraud. It is troubling to learn that 12% of the audits of scientific studies conducted by the U.S. Food and Drug Administration from 1977 to 1985 revealed serious deficiencies; studies conducted after 1985 had a somewhat lower percentage of deficiencies (Shapiro and Charrow 1989). Considering the importance of scientific work, including medical drug evaluations, this level of fraud and deceit is significant in its possible effect on health and the expense of scientific research.

Surprisingly, scientific deceit is not just a contemporary problem. Modern analyses of the data of historical scientific giants such as the physicist Isaac Newton and the father of modern genetics, Gregor Mendel, indicate that they "fudged" data in an effort to promulgate their theories. Charles Darwin appears to have "borrowed" to a considerable extent from the intellectual work of scientists who preceded him, yet he did not give them due credit. American Nobel prize laureate Robert Millikan used data only from those experiments that supported his theories. This "cooking" of his data allowed him to defeat his rival Felix Ehrenhaft, who, in retrospect, may have been more accurate in his conceptualization of the electronic charge (Broad and Wade 1982).

Even the nineteenth-century giant of French medicine, Louis Pasteur, was not "immune" to deceit. A recent study of Pasteur's notebooks revealed that on several occasions he violated the medical and scientific ethical standards that he advocated (C. Anderson 1993). In one famous experiment, he used a vaccine created by a technique of a competitor while claiming he had created it by his own methods. Pasteur's competitor, a veterinarian named Toussaint, had a nervous breakdown and died a few months after Pasteur's highly successful and internationally acclaimed trial of the vaccine.

There is little doubt at this time that the "research" of Sir Cyril Burt, for which he was knighted, was forged. He had claimed to relate the intelligence quotient (IQ) to social class and, as a result, influenced social-educational policies in Britain. A brilliant man, Burt was regarded by many as the preeminent psychologist in the United Kingdom, and through his editorship of a major psychology journal, he was able to influence and shape opinions and to suppress criticism (D. J. Miller and Hersen 1992).

During the past two decades, several dramatic cases of scientific fraud have received wide publicity. Among these are the experiments of Mark Spector at Cornell University. Spector produced experiments that purified new enzymes and led quickly to a new and exciting theory of the cause of cancer—the *kinase cascade*. However, the experiments could not be replicated and later proved to be forged, as were his academic degrees (and checks he wrote for nearly $5,000). The check forgeries resulted in a suspended prison sentence. Spector's behavior was most embarrassing to his supervisor, Efraim Racker, and to Cornell University (D. J. Miller and Hersen 1992).

Similarly embarrassing to Harvard University and to Eugene Braunwald, a distinguished cardiologist, was the discovery that a bright young academic star, John Darsee, had forged experiments while he was in Boston and also during his earlier work at other institutions (D. J. Miller and Hersen 1992).

At yet another Ivy League school, Yale, it was determined that Dr. Vigay R. Soman, who had come to the United States from India, plagiarized research papers that were in the process of review and published the results as his own. This process was facilitated by his use of the name of a distinguished professor of medicine, Dr. Phillip Filig, as a coauthor. Discovery of the ruse was not only embarrassing to Filig but also caused Filig to lose a prestigious endowed chair at another university. The offer to Filig was withdrawn when news of the scandal became widely known (Broad 1980a, 1980b).

Although these and similar cases have generated considerable publicity, they may represent only the tip of the iceberg. D. J. Miller and Hersen (1992) believe that fraud in the sciences is more widespread than is generally acknowledged. During my own career in academic medicine, I have repeatedly witnessed incidents or heard stories of various forms of fraud, data theft, or outright plagiarism.

The pressures on today's young scientists are immense. They must "publish or perish." But even the publication of a respectable number of papers is not sufficient. Promotions and tenure now depend on the procurement of funding from outside sources. Thus, the young scientist must *quickly* come up with some positive findings (negative findings have a low value for potential publication) and convince a funding agency to grant money to continue the research. Busy senior investigators—overwhelmed with their own career pressures—frequently are absent, provide little supervision to younger collaborators, and put their names on poorly supervised scientific works to provide the papers with more credibility and to advance their own careers by adding to their curricula vitae.

In scientific fraud, the risk of discovery is relatively low, and the process of review (even in the best peer-reviewed journals) may not detect scientifically flawed or fraudulent research. This is particularly true when all of the important data are not included in the paper (Rennie 1989). Authors are encouraged to keep their communication short and crisp. Thus, only relevant data are selected to present for publication. However, conscious or unconscious motivation may serve to select only those data that support the author(s)' conclusions. The current academic climate fosters temptation, capitulation of scientific values, and opportunities to engage in deceitful behavior.

Psychologists are not exempt from deceit, and the research techniques of experimental psychology often use deception in one form or another. Such deception may potentially harm subjects and give them false ideas about themselves (e.g., "Our test reveals that you exhibit homosexual tendencies") (Toy et al. 1989). Menger (1973) reviewed the frequency of the use of deception as an experimental technique in published psychological research. He found that the frequency varied from 3.1% of the papers published in one journal to 47.2% of the papers in the *Journal of Personality and Social Psychology* (JPSP). A decade later—*after* the adoption of ethical regulations for psychological research—the percentage of published papers that involved deception as a research technique had actually increased to 58.5% in JPSP (Adair et al. 1985).

All in all, the evidence suggests that scientists, who by definition search for truth, are not immune from the use of deceit in their experimental techniques or in their reports of their results. One senior scientist (Branscomb 1985) cautions that the problem in science stems not so much from overt fraud but rather from self-deception. Scientists, in their wish to publish results, often gloss over data, do not review their work for the possibility of systemic errors, and fail to state the contributions of others appropriately.

Developing a Psychology of Deceit

America's increasing interest in the subject of deceit is reflected in the recent publication of a number of books dealing with lying or including the word "lie" (or its synonyms) in the title: *A Bright and Shining Lie* (Sheehan 1988); *People of the Lie* (Peck 1983); *Lying: Moral Choice in Public and Private Life* (Bok 1978a); *The Penguin Books of Lies* (Kerr 1990); *The Dance of Deception* (Lerner 1993); *Private Lies* (Pittman 1989); the previously noted *The Day America Told the Truth* (Patterson and Kim 1991); *Telling Lies* (Ekman 1992); and *Vital Lies, Simple Truths* (Goleman 1985). Scholarly efforts have also been made to understand some aspects of the psychology of lying and self-deception: *The Varnished Truth* (Nyberg 1993); *Self-Deception: An Adaptive Mechanism?* (Lockard and Paulus 1988); *Deception: Perspectives on Human and Nonhuman Deceit* (Mitchell and Thompson 1986); *Lying and Deception in Everyday Life* (M. Lewis and Saarni 1993); and *The Prevalence of Deceit* (Bailey 1991). These excellent books have examined some issues of deceit, but each has focused on limited aspects of deceit, thereby narrowing its approach to the subject.

In this book, I approach the subject of deceit in an admittedly ambitious attempt to be comprehensive, and I investigate the phenomena of both "normal" and "pathological" deceit. My perspective is that of a clinical psychiatrist who has frequently worked with pathological liars. I have tried to separate the issue of morality from the subject matter. Complete adherence to that goal is obviously impossible, and despite the best of intentions, some of my biases will inevitably show through.

The vignettes at the opening of this chapter—all actual occurrences—and the descriptions of lying in everyday life, the workplace, politics, medicine, and science illustrate the widely varied aspects of lying. It is a truism, but important to acknowledge, that there are different types of lies, different types of liars, and different situations in which lies are told. Every lie has a predisposing condition, and because most are perpetuated within a social situation, these social factors influence the telling of the lie, its content, and the response to it.

It is intriguing that some people compulsively lie even when "the truth would serve them better." Why? Also, some people lie despite their wishes and attempts to be truthful. Some preliminary evidence suggests that specific forms of brain dysfunction influence such behaviors. Furthermore, as I explore in this book, the most common form of deceit is probably self-deception. Why would one lie to oneself, and doesn't the term sound like an oxymoron? In fact, lying to others and to oneself are much more closely linked than one might suspect on first glance.

This exploration of the psychology of deceit begins by examining the language of lying. The English language is rich in words to describe various forms of prevarication. It is instructive to review the various classifications of deceit that have been proposed.

After clarifying the terminology of lying, I investigate deceit from a biological perspective. Deceitful behaviors are common in lower animals and primates. It has been suggested, in fact, that deceitful behavior is one of the variables that is intrinsic to survival and that influences the outcomes of evolution through differential reproduction. In reference to biological substrates of behavior, the brain, which is the site of information processing, both input and output, must also be considered. The brain has the capacity to consciously distort the output of information (deceiving others) but also to distort input (deceiving oneself). The structure and function of the brain, influenced by both genetic and pathological or disease factors, determine the characteristics of information processing and the various mechanisms of deceit. Medical and neurological data indicate that brain dysfunction is an important contributor to pathological lying in some individuals.

Regardless of how brain structure may influence information processing and pathological lying in some individuals, it remains a fact that everybody lies. The process of psychological development is closely related to how we learn to communicate or miscommunicate with both ourselves and others. As we progress through childhood, we are taught not only the skills associated with successful lying but also when and where to lie. Lying becomes an essential component of the process of individuation (i.e., the establishment of personal autonomy and comfortable interpersonal relationships). Woe to the "pathological truth-teller" who does not know how to keep his or her mouth shut!

In the exploration of why people lie, we will learn that there are many different reasons that any one lie gets told. Greed, wish fulfillment, sadistic impulses, and the need to bolster one's self-esteem are among these complex motives. Perhaps the most important reason that people lie, however, is that the lie facilitates self-deception; people lie to others in order to lie to themselves. Not only do they lie to themselves but they encourage others to lie to them in order to reinforce their self-deception. Thus, the process of lying and self-deception becomes intimately interwoven with a basic ego mechanism: reality testing.

In this regard, we discover that memory is more malleable than previously believed and that through another person's lies or misrepresentations, a person may come to have false memories. This, in association with self-deception, may result in false accusations and false confessions.

It is not surprising to learn that people lie and deceive themselves in individually characteristic manners. Often such a pattern can be identified as one of the clinically described personality traits or disorders. In traditional psychoanalytic terms, a "hysteric" uses lying to assist with repression and to obtain approval from others, whereas an "obsessive" uses deception to maintain autonomy and control. People who abuse alcohol and other chemical substances are frequently skilled liars; they lie both to hide their behavior and to deceive themselves.

Lying and deception may be so pervasive for an individual that they take over much of that person's life. People who have factitious disorder (Munchausen syndrome) represent an extreme example; these people spend most of their energy in fooling physicians and other health care professionals. A similar and closely related syndrome is *imposture*—a fascinating phenomenon that is the subject of popular books and movies and of serious scrutiny by psychiatrists.

Successful impostors and con artists are obviously bright, talented, and filled with potential for genuine personal accomplishment. Yet they seem compelled not only to tell lies but to live a lie.

If—and there really seems to be little doubt—we live in a world that thrives on deception, the individual must learn how to sort through a constant bombardment of information to determine its accuracy. Just as a child learns how to lie, the child must also learn how to "read" others and make decisions about the veracity of communications. For some individuals, such as police officers, customs inspectors, and poker players, learning how to detect deception becomes a life's work. At times, mechanical devices (e.g., lie detectors) are used with the belief (perhaps mistaken) that they will assist in determining the truth.

Are the effects of lying always bad, as implied by the moralizing of parents, institutions, and the Pinocchio myth? Hardly. If lying always had negative consequences, we would all be stumbling over our noses daily. Lies are advantageously used by individuals and social groups to obtain power, sexual gratification, and material goods or wealth. It is also likely that a person's ability to read another person's need for self-deception—and to satisfy those needs—is highly associated with skills for careers in sales and politics. For most people, the skill for self-deception is closely related to the skill for deceiving others and may also be correlated with a sense of well-being and confidence for facing the future in an uncertain world.

Summary

Lying and self-deception permeate all aspects of human life and social interactions. Societal messages about deceit are often contradictory; we teach our children how to lie effectively and encourage others to lie to us even as we condemn lying as a vice. The development of a comprehensive psychology of deceit must consider these paradoxes in addition to the biological, intrapsychic, and societal influences on the process of human deception.

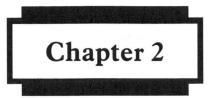

Chapter 2

Defining Deceit: The Language of Lying

Man was given a tongue with which to speak and words to hide his thoughts.

—Hungarian proverb

The full genius of language is inseparable from the impulse to concealment and fiction.

—Steiner

The language of lying is often complex and confusing, reflecting the nature of the subject itself. Deception occurs by a variety of means, some with conscious intent and others without. To lie is, by definition, to be deceptive, but not all forms of deception are lying. In this chapter, I consider the various definitions of lying and its associated permutations, the use of nonverbal communication to deceive, and some of the language used to describe the phenomenon of self-deception.

Lying: Deceiving Others

Webster's Seventh New Collegiate Dictionary (1971) defines "to lie" as 1) to assert something known or believed by the speaker to be untrue with intent to deceive, or 2) to create a false or misleading impression. This commonly accepted definition contains two major components. The first is the statement of something believed to be untrue by the liar (the content of the lie), and the second is motivation, the intent to deceive. Interestingly, the definition does not specify "words" but rather the intent to create a false impression. In popular usage, and even among psychologists working in this area of research, a "lie" usually refers to words alone.

The misrepresentations of a psychotic person are not considered to be lies because the person believes them. Nor do we consider honest mistakes or statements made on the basis of misinformation to be lies. Thus, we can have a situation in which deliberately false information (a lie) is passed from one person to a second who believes it. The same information is then passed from the second person to a third person. This secondary transmission of the original lie would not be considered a lie, even though the content of the misinformation is the same for both statements.

As simple as the above definition appears to be, it does lead to some fascinating paradoxes. For instance, it is possible to tell the truth and yet have the intent to deceive (half of the practical definition of lying). For example, a secretary explains to her superior that she is 30 minutes late to work because there had been a terrible accident on the interstate highway. She was technically correct, but she told only part of the truth. In fact, the accident was on the other side of the highway on which she was traveling, and it delayed her only a minute or two. By telling only half the truth, she had effectively deceived.

In yet another situation, one may tell "the truth" but may lie! If one incorrectly believes something to be true and deliberately states the opposite (which *is* true) in an effort to deceive, then the full definition of lying has been met because of the intent to deceive, even though the truth was spoken.

Language of Lying

The English language has many terms and euphemisms to describe lying (see Table 2–1). Karpman (1953) commented that the number of synonyms for "truth" is small, but those related to lying might fill several pages in a dictionary. Shibles (1985) noted that a rich vocabulary of deceit is not unique to English and provided a long list of German words descriptive of lying. "Lying" is a remarkably emotional word, and to accuse a person of being a "liar" is regarded as an attack. To call someone a liar might, in some cultures, be tantamount to a challenge for a duel. The use of euphemisms softens the aggressive nature of words referring to deceit and also provides gradations of culpability. I define and briefly discuss a few of these words.

Table 2–1. Examples of words that connote deceit

Verbs	Nouns	Adjectives
Belie	Affectation	Clandestine
Bluff	Canard	Double-dealing
Cant	Casuistry	Sham
Cheat	Dishonesty	Surreptitious
Conceal	Disinformation	Untruthful
Connive	Dissimulation	
Contrive	Double-face	
Counterfeit	Duplicity	
Deceive	Fallacy	
Defraud	False-hearted	
Dissemble	Falsehood	
Exaggerate	Fraud	
Fabricate	Humbug	
Fake	Hypocrisy	
Feign	Perfidy	
Fib	Pretension	
Impersonate	Sophistry	
Lie	Stealth	
Malinger	Treachery	
Misrepresent	Trickery	
Perjure	Understatement	
Plagiarize		
Pretend		
Prevaricate		
Slander		

Prevarication means deviation from the truth. It is derived from the Latin term meaning to walk crookedly. To *perjure* oneself is to voluntarily (knowingly) provide false statements while under oath. A *fib* is a lie, but it implies one that is trivial or childish. A *mendacious* person is characterized by deception or falsehood. Two words frequently used by historians are *dissemble* and *ingenuous*. The former means to put on a false appearance—to conceal facts, feelings, or intentions. The latter suggests showing a childlike simplicity or naivete, but with a hint of a self-deceptive quality.

New words periodically creep into usage, which are probably attempts to soften the emotional impact of words such as *lies* or *liar*. During the Reagan administration, the word "disinformation" emerged as a description of deliberate misinformation. During the Iran-Contra investigation, witnesses "groped for polite ways to say the L word. They have confessed to having told half-truths (as opposed to half-lies), or having told the literal truth instead of the real truth." (Baldwin 1989, p. 35). Euphemisms for lying are not limited to American politicians. Winston Churchill used "terminological inexactitude" to describe deceit, and a subsequent British government employed "an economy of the truth" to describe its deceptions (W. P. Robinson 1993).

Levels of Lying

Lies differ in their complexity and sophistication. Leekam (1992) proposed three levels of lying. She describes the first level as manipulating the behavior of another person without the intent (or even the idea) of influencing the other's beliefs. Leekam suggests that such lies are told by small children who may deny misbehaviors to avoid punishment or falsely claim to have done something good to get a reward. These are generally "learned" strategies, employed without understanding that saying something untrue can affect the listener's beliefs. Obviously, these simple lies often fail because small children tend to lie at the wrong time or neglect important issues such as covering their tracks (e.g., leaving cookie crumbs).

The second level of lying takes into account the liar's awareness of the listener's beliefs. The liar must now keep in mind that the false statement (lie) may manipulate the listener's beliefs, that the listener will evaluate the statement as being true or false, and that the listener will, on the basis of the new belief (if the lie has been accepted), evaluate future statements in the light of the new belief. Liars who have reached this level of developmental sophistication are much more effective at deception than are first-level liars. For example, a car salesperson may size up a customer and be deceitful as to certain attributes (e.g., fuel economy, safety, or reliability record) of the car that he or she is selling.

On reaching the third level of lying competence, the liar recognizes not only the effect of the words spoken on the listener's beliefs but also that the listener may be evaluating the liar's own beliefs about the words. In other words, how sincere is the liar? Thus, skilled lying involves convincing the listener that the speaker believes what he or she is saying and has a truthful intention. A skilled liar also continuously "reads" the listener's nonverbal behavior and, in response to "feedback" from the listener, adjusts both verbal and nonverbal communications to be more credible. This skill markedly enhances one's capacity to manipulate other peoples' beliefs and behaviors. Leekam suggests that this ability may be the hallmark of subtle acts of tact, persuasion, and diplomacy. An example of this skill is that the aforementioned car salesperson could "read" the effect of his or her sales pitch on the potential customer. If any disbelief were detected, the salesperson would immediately alter his or her behavior to appear more sincere and credible.

These levels of lying are developmental steps that are not mastered by all people, although most people can learn to lie at the second level.

There is yet another level of skill at other-deception that we can term *advanced lying*. Relatively few persons achieve this sophistication in deceit, but among those that do are certain charismatic politicians, evangelists, sales professionals, poker players, and con artists. These persons, especially the con artists (see Chapter 8), use psychological ploys to quickly convince their "marks" of their complete trustworthiness, even to the point that life's savings may be handed over to almost complete strangers. Persons with these skills have mastered techniques of monitoring their own nonverbal behavior and controlling it as a means of conscious communication that is simultaneous with their speech.

One politician was notably skillful at dissembling and controlling his nonverbal messages. He always made it a point to make only positive comments about anyone. If, however, he wanted the listener to think poorly of another person, he would provide subtle nonverbal hints of disgust while extolling the person's virtues. The message being broadcast was: "I am really a nice person who likes everybody, but this guy is really a sleazeball." Predictably, some of the people discredited by this manipulative politician were actually fine, upright, and decent people who were slandered through deceptive nonverbal communication (see section, "Nonverbal Deceit," later in this chapter).

Classification of Lies

The existence of numerous terms for lying suggests the need in the English language to differentiate various, perhaps subtle, distinctions of the types of lies. Some authors have also classified lies into separate categories depending on the malignancy, personal psychopathology of the liar, and target of the lie (Bok 1978a; Davidoff 1942; Karpman 1953). Such classifications must be viewed with caution because they may have moral implications. Table 2–2 provides one such classification.

Different types of lies. The terminology used to classify lies is often obvious. However, it may also be subject to individual or idiosyncratic interpretation. Some commonly used terms are described below.

White lies are basically social lies that serve to lubricate interpersonal relationships. They are frequently provided in such an automatic manner as not even to register in consciousness. For example,

▌ "I enjoyed your party. Thank you so much for inviting me." (The truth is that the invitation was accepted because of occupational necessity, and the party was deadly boring.)

▌ "I'm sorry that I can't go out with you Saturday night. I have a previous engagement." (The truth is that the girl wouldn't be "caught dead" in public with the nerd who is asking her for a date, and the previous engagement is washing her hair.)

▋ "I'm fine. How are you?" in response to "Hi. How are you today?" from a salesclerk. (The truth is that the person has a terrible headache and under the best of circumstances couldn't care less about the health of a stranger.)

In general, white lies are social conventions that convey little intention to deceive. They primarily serve to respect the sensitivity and dignity of others. Yet many persons regard any lie as morally reprehensible and will strive to make their statements as factually accurate as possible, sometimes by telling only a portion of the truth. For example, in the first situation, the individual might reword the thanks to: "I really appreciate it that you thought enough of us to invite us to your party."

Humorous lies are those aimed at amusing the listener, and any intent to deceive is transient and teasing. Characteristically, they involve some degree of preposterous exaggeration. For example,

▋ "Oh, darling! We are so happy to be at your party. When we received your invitation, we interrupted our vacation in Monte Carlo and immediately flew back." (This statement was made by

Table 2–2. A classification of lying

Type of lie	Motive
Benign and salutary lies	To effect social conventions
Hysterical lies	To attract attention
Defensive lies	To extricate oneself from a difficult situation
Compensatory lies	To impress another person
Malicious lies	To deceive for personal gain
Gossip	To exaggerate rumors maliciously
Implied lies	To mislead by partial truths
"Love intoxication" lies	To exaggerate idealistically
Pathological lies	To lie self-destructively

Source.   Adapted from Karpman B: "Lying," in *Encyclopedia of Aberrations: A Psychiatric Handbook.* Edited by Podolsky E. New York, Philosophical Library, 1953, pp. 288–300.

a neighbor who was invited to a backyard barbecue.)

▪ "I sold so much dog food last week that no horse within 50 miles was safe." (This statement was made by a sales manager for a dog-food company.)

Altruistic lies are those lies that are told to benefit someone else, to reduce suffering, or to help increase self-esteem. The most commonly cited altruistic lies are those told by professionals to persons for whom they are caring. For example,

▪ "Mrs. Jones, you don't have anything to worry about. We will have this cancer licked with chemotherapy." (This was told to a woman with widespread metastatic ovarian cancer.)
▪ "I know that it's painful now, but you will be united with her in Heaven." (This statement was made by a hospital chaplain to a couple whose daughter had just died of a cocaine overdose.)
▪ "Of course you are attractive, and there is someone who will want to marry you." (This statement was made by the mother of an unattractive and borderline mentally retarded teenage daughter.)

Although the ostensible purpose of the altruistic lie is to serve the needs of the person to whom the lie is told, such lies may actually be motivated by the lying person's discomfort with the situation (Bok 1978b).

Defensive lies are those told to protect oneself and others. They may be told to avoid punishment or attack from others or to preserve self-esteem. For example,

▪ "No, I didn't get into the cookie jar." (This was said to a mother by her 4-year-old son who had chocolate smeared on his face.)
▪ "There is no one here except our family members." (This was told to German Gestapo agents by a Dutch family hiding Jews during World War II.)
▪ "I don't know what happened. All of a sudden the computer malfunctioned." (This was said by a secretary who accidentally deleted an entire file, an essential manuscript, from her computer's hard drive memory.)

Defensive lies are among those that are easiest to understand and perhaps justify. People who lie to protect themselves or others are acting in self-defense, a time-honored behavior. A lie told in defense of others may also be seen as altruistic.

Aggressive lies are told in an effort to hurt someone else or to gain an advantage for oneself. For example,

- "... and he was so cheap, he wouldn't buy me dinner!" (This was told to friends by a young woman who was angry that a man had not asked her out for a second date.)
- "I type 60 words per minute." (This was told by an applicant for a receptionist job. Her actual typing rate was 40 words per minute with multiple errors.)
- "Our ships in the Tonkin Gulf were attacked last night by forces of the North Vietnamese Navy." (This was told by the president of the United States to obtain approval for bombing attacks on Hanoi. No evidence of such an attack was ever discovered.)

Aggressive lies are self-serving and may potentially damage others, and therefore, most people would see them as clearly immoral.

Pathological lies (compulsive lies) are of special interest to persons studying the psychology of lying. As used in this book, pathological lies are those that are told even when there is little or no apparent gain to the person who is lying. In fact, the lying often occurs even when the results would be better if the truth were told. Furthermore, the lie is not determined solely by situational factors and appears to be compulsive or fantastic (Selling 1942). In general, lies are termed pathological when they interfere with normal development or are destructive to the quality of the life of the person who tells the lie.

Pseudologia fantastica is a specific form of pathological lying in which the pseudologue (the liar) tells involved stories about life circumstances, both present and past (King and Ford 1988). At first, the stories may seem believable, but with time the inconsistencies often betray their fantastic qualities. Detecting the falsehood is often difficult because there may be a skillful blending of fact and fantasy. The stories are told as if they were real, and the person's emotional state may be consistent with the content provided, thereby supporting the story's apparent authenticity. For example, one pseudologue told the convincing story, while weeping genuine tears, of a car wreck that killed his fiancée and her two young children. The entire story was later proved to be a fabrication. A Munchausen patient who was simulating chest pain claimed to be a commercial airline pilot. He stated that because of pain, while landing at Detroit, he had to turn the controls over to his copilot. He further stated that as an Air Force pilot during World War II he had been forced to eject from his burning plane and received shrapnel injuries. In fact, this "patient" was not a pilot, but he did have a police record of 33 arrests and convictions for forgery, alcohol-related disturbances, and other misdemeanors (Heym 1973). Examples of pathological lies (and liars) and pseudologia fantastica are described in Chapters 7 and 8.

When vigorously confronted with their fabrications, pseudologues can acknowledge that they are not true, thereby demonstrating that the stories are not the delusional products of a psychotic person. However, in their explanations of the discrepancies, they may (convincingly) provide new fabrications. Attempting to determine the "truth" from these persons is like trying to catch a greased pig.

Secrets

A secret is something known by one or more persons but deliberately hidden from one or more other persons. Thus, a secret may involve either one person or many. Secrets are often closely related to lies (Pittman 1989). By withholding information, the secretholder may knowingly create false beliefs in others. For example, a man does not tell his wife that he has been fired from his job and continues to get up and leave the house each morning; he thereby falsely maintains her belief that he is working. Maintaining a secret often requires lying; it may involve self-deception in that the person allows himself or herself to consider only the protective function of the secret (Lerner 1993).

Secrets serve to maintain privacy (regarded to be a legitimate right by Bok [1983] but not by the totalitarian state in the book *1984* by Orwell [1949]) and also to support the functions of a group.

Shared secrets increase bonding, maintain cohesiveness, and protect family or organizational structure (Vangelisti 1994). For example, a family may maintain secrecy about the alcoholism of a parent in an effort to maintain the appearance of normalcy. When a family has many secrets, particularly secrets involving more than one family member (e.g., incest), dissatisfaction grows among family members, resulting in a dysfunctional family (Vangelisti 1994). As discussed in Chapters 6 and 13, intimacy requires honest communication and a shared base of knowledge, which are obviously impaired by keeping secrets.

Nonverbal Deceit

Communication is not limited to the words we use. Humans also communicate by a variety of nonverbal means, including the emotions displayed (or concealed) and characteristic symbolic gestures (emblems; see Chapter 10) (H. G. Johnson et al. 1975). For example, every adult American knows what it means to "give someone the finger." These nonverbal communications may stand on their own as messages or serve as metacommunications to modify the verbal messages being delivered. Affect (emotional display) can be used to emphasize a verbal statement or to negate it (Ekman and Friesen 1969a). Furthermore, just as one can use words to deceive, one can also use nonverbal channels of communication to deceive. Skilled liars, as noted earlier in this chapter, have some measure of control over their nonverbal behavior and expression of emotions.

B. M. DePaulo (1988) suggests that nonverbal deceit is more common than many people realize. Such deceit may be difficult to articulate in words or store into memory simply because it is nonverbal. An example of nonverbal deceit was provided by C. R. Snyder and Higgins (1988). A baseball pitcher whose pitches were being hit by the other team was pulled from the game by his manager. As he left the mound, he began rubbing his pitching arm. The nonverbal message was: "I'm really not that bad of a pitcher. I have a sore arm today." Simulation of physical symptoms may be a common form of nonverbal deceit.

Four major strategies can be used to modify nonverbal behavior: minimization, exaggeration, neutralization, and substitution of emotions and behaviors (Ekman and Friesen 1969a; Saarni 1982).

Minimization. The result of an individual's attempt to dampen the external appearance of a more deeply experienced emotion is minimization of emotional expression. For example, a surgeon whose patient is failing rapidly after an operation may present himself to the family as "concerned" but outwardly calm, while inwardly he feels panicky as he perceives the looming disaster.

Exaggeration. Maximization of felt emotions reflects a dramatic attempt to influence another person. Saarni (1982) suggests that this nonverbal deceit may be the first type of deceit to emerge developmentally. Children are more likely to cry after experiencing a minor injury when they believe that they are being observed than when they believe that no one is attending to them. Persons with a histrionic personality style (see Chapter 6) are more likely to exaggerate their emotions in an attention-seeking manner.

Neutralization. An effort to mask emotional response by adapting a "poker face" is known as neutralization. Psychoanalysts and other professionals may display relatively little response in their efforts to appear nonjudgmental of the patient's or client's statements. Ekman and Friesen (1974) contend, however, that it is difficult to maintain strict neutrality of emotion and that one's true emotions tend to leak out.

Substitution. A common mechanism of hiding one's true feelings is substitution of emotions. One of the most common techniques employed for this purpose is to substitute "pleasure" for a negative emotion. Smiling is one of the easiest nonverbal communications to produce and may be used to mask feelings of arrogance, anxiety, or boredom (Ekman et al. 1988). A shopkeeper may keep smiling even when he or she wishes that a demanding customer, who is unlikely to make a purchase, would leave the store. An employee may smile and graciously accept constructive criticism from a supervisor, even when he or she feels it is unjust.

The importance of nonverbal behavior is so great that no study of deceit can be intelligently pursued without considering this channel of communication.

Self-Deception: Lying to Oneself

Self-deception at first glance seems to be a contradiction in terms. How can one not know that which one knows? Yet the concept of self-deception is well established in common language (e.g., "you know in your heart that . . .") and has been explored by both psychoanalysts and experimental psychologists. Furthermore, the phenomena of hallucinations and delusions in a psychotic person are concrete evidence for self-deception.

Dr. Anthony Greenwald (1980), a psychologist who is now at the University of Washington, has provided a provocative view of how the executive portion of a person's mind (i.e., the "ego") functions in a manner similar to that of a totalitarian state as depicted in Orwell's *1984*. In Greenwald's view, the flow of information is kept under very tight control, and deceptive (self-deceptive in terms of the individual) techniques may be used in this process. Greenwald suggests that the individual has the cognitive bias of egocentricity; that is, one's self is the focus of knowledge. An individual tends to see himself or herself as responsible for desired outcomes but not for undesired ones. Thus, there is resistance to new or different information, which may be selectively ignored (cognitive conservatism). Greenwald speculates that those self-deceptive mechanisms help the individual to organize knowledge and maintain goals and to avoid being overwhelmed by the continuing inflow of new, potentially ambiguous or psychologically conflictive information.

Concepts of the Unconscious

To understand the concept of self-deception, we must assume that some functions of mental activity occur outside conscious awareness. Unconscious processes are evident in many of our activities that at one time required conscious effort but were learned and can now be repeated by rote, without conscious awareness (e.g., playing a memorized piece on a musical instrument). We do not, however, speak of playing an instrument as self-deception just because it is an automatic activity. To deceive oneself implies that at least two simultaneous ideas in one's brain are related to the same issue but are contradictory. Self-deception involves maintaining one idea in one's consciousness while suppressing another conflicting idea. Furthermore, people may, at different times, act in a motivated manner on one or the other of their beliefs (Gur and Sackheim 1979). Thus, one must often self-deceive to maintain psychic equilibrium.

The evidence for mental activity outside consciousness is quite robust and has been superbly outlined by Dr. Daniel Goleman (1985) in his book *Vital Lies, Simple Truths.* Goleman provides various hypothetical models of mental activity and research findings that support these concepts. He concludes that the large majority of mental activity occurs outside of consciousness. Stored memories, both conscious and unconscious, are dynamically involved to preserve psychic equilibrium. Among the unconscious mental activities is an "intelligent filter" that controls the perception, storage, and retrieval of information. Some things that are "seen" may not be perceived and therefore not stored.

Few psychologists or psychiatrists would question the existence of the unconscious. The current issue does not appear to be whether there is an unconscious, but how to explain consciousness (Horgan 1994). However, the characteristics and functions of the unconscious remain an issue for debate; is the unconscious smart or dumb (Loftus and Klinger 1992)? There seems to be little doubt that unconscious mechanisms influence perception and are capable of processing multidimensional and interactive relationships of different forms of information (Lewicki et al. 1992). This mechanism of information processing may explain why some individuals are remarkably intuitive—one type of intelligence. Greenwald (1992) suggested that the unconscious is a type of infrastructure network for information processing but doubted that it is capable of the sophisticated cognitive logic attributed to it by psychoanalysts. A different, more encompassing view was offered by Erdelyi (1992), who did not reject the concept of Greenwald's network model of unconscious cognition, but suggested that this model is consistent with complex internal processes, including the defense mechanisms (see below) or schemata (chunks of [mis]information that connote attitudes, such as all men are exploitative or all women are manipulative) that can be activated without access to conscious verbal processes.

My view of the unconscious is similar to that of Erdelyi. To use the computer analogy, many of our cognitive functions (information processing) are like a software program—devoid of content per se, but directing the input and use of new information. In addition, some information may be stored that is not readily accessible to conscious control. Clinicians who have seen repressed memories emerge believe in this process, whereas scientists, who cannot experimentally reproduce it in the laboratory, continue to express doubts. An example from my clinical experience occurred while I was conducting an Amytal interview (the so-called truth serum) of a young woman who had been assaulted during a robbery; her companion had been murdered. She had sustained a head injury and could not remember any details surrounding the incident. In a drugged state, the woman clearly identified the assailant as an acquaintance, emotionally stating that she "couldn't believe" that he was capable of such an act. Based on this lead, an investigation provided evidence that the suspect had committed the crime, and he subsequently confessed. His conviction was based on collaborative evidence, not the Amytal interview. One process of excluding unwelcome memories from consciousness is called *dissociation* (see below). (For alternative views of recovered memories, see Chapter 9.)

There is growing evidence that neuroanatomical or physiological factors may play an important role in the compartmentalizing of thoughts and feelings. Thus, in a very concrete fashion (again using computer terminology), conflicting data may be stored in different "files" that do not interact with one another. (See Chapter 3 in reference to "split-brain" patients.) One tenable hypothesis is that some psychological functions may be responsible for the "switching" that makes various areas of stored memories available at different times.

The traditional psychoanalytic model postulates that many of one's conscious thoughts, feelings, and behaviors are determined by unconscious influences. Much of this influence is exerted through various ego-defense mechanisms. Ego-defense mechanisms promote psychological equilibrium by defending the individual from painful or conflictive thoughts and feelings that cause anxiety. By reflecting and transforming reality information, they help regulate self-esteem and modulate emotional responses. As such, and to the extent that they do not massively interfere with reality testing, they are adaptive and serve as coping mechanisms (Cramer 1987).

Ego-Defense Mechanisms

Ego-defense mechanisms were originally described by Anna Freud (1936/1966). Not all psychologists and psychiatrists accept psychoanalytic concepts and the idea of an active unconscious. However, D. W. Hamlyn (1985, p. 210), a professor of philosophy at the University of London, acknowledges that "the concept of self-deception is close to the Freudian or psychoanalytic concept of repression."

Ego-defense mechanisms are phenomena that are easily recognized and identified without a need to tie them to a particular theoretical perspective. They are descriptions of mental processes, not explanations, and therefore do not require a psychoanalytic perspective; they can also be explained using learning theory. I propose that a common feature of each of these defense mechanisms is that they assist in the process of self-deception. Regardless of the terminology, these are the means by which we fool ourselves.

The following descriptions of various ego-defense mechanisms are limited to those that are common and those that do not require a specific theoretical bias to understand or interpret. The descriptions follow, to a large extent, the classification by Vaillant and colleagues (Vaillant 1971; Vaillant et al. 1986). Any behavior or psychic mechanism can usually be interpreted as reflecting one or more of these mechanisms. They are often used in clusters; for example, intellectualization is closely related to isolation, rationalization, and reaction formation.

Denial represents a rejection of reality and of facts that are readily verified. It can be identified in adolescents who engage in reckless, life-threatening behavior and who may deny that anything could happen to them, as well as in people who ignore symptoms of illness. For example, a woman ignored a hard and growing lump in her breast until the skin decomposed and the foul-smelling discharge directed her daughter's attention to her condition.

Delusional projection refers to frank delusions about external reality. Internal needs massively distort reality. For example, a man whose own sexual behavior made him feel guilty transformed this guilt and anxiety into a belief that his wife had been unfaithful. In his ensuing rage over her imagined behavior, he might have attacked or even killed her. In another case, a middle-aged woman became convinced that her psychiatrist was in love with her. She followed him, became angry when he was with his wife (interpreting this as infidelity), and even called the wife to inform her that the psychiatrist would be filing for divorce in order to remarry. The entire episode represented a delusional projection of the patient's infatuation with her psychiatrist. This particular syndrome is well known and has been labeled the *de Clerambault syndrome,* for the French psychiatrist who first identified it.

Distortion involves grossly reshaping external reality to meet one's inner needs. Distortion may sometimes be associated with internal religious beliefs and, as such, may be adaptive. A devoutly religious woman dying of lymphoma remained unperturbed and stated calmly that she knew that her faith in "the Master" would reverse the disease process.

Projection is the process of attributing one's own unacknowledged thoughts or feelings to another person. A secretary loudly protested that she had no interest in the friend of a co-worker's fiancé and that she would not date him. When asked if he had ever approached her for a date, she admitted that he had not. Projection is a common mechanism seen frequently in day-to-day life. For example, a wife accused her husband of being angry, when, in truth, she was the one who was angry, but she could not acknowledge her feelings.

Acting out describes behavior that is initiated from poorly modulated anxiety or instinctive drives. Persons with antisocial and borderline personality disorders are notably impulsive and are more likely to engage in acting-out behaviors. Examples of such behavior are sexual impulses, which may result in promiscuity; aggressive impulses, which may result in violent acts; and anxiety or depression, which may result in substance abuse or self-mutilation.

Hypochondriasis describes the transformation of reproach or anger toward other persons into reproach toward oneself and then into perceptions of pain and other physical symptoms (Vaillant 1971). A clinical illustration is that of a middle-aged woman who developed hypochondriacal symptoms after her youngest child married and left home. The woman felt lonely and abandoned, not only by her children but also by her husband, who was preoccupied with business endeavors and golf. Her symptoms represented unconscious (self-deceptive) attempts to deny her anger and, simultaneously through the induction of guilt, to manipulate her husband and children to care for her.

Passive-aggressive behavior describes turning aggression in toward oneself. It often involves hurting oneself or engaging in self-defeating behavior in an effort to make others feel guilty or to defeat their wishes. A young man, whose parents had repeatedly expressed their wishes for his academic success, failed out of many colleges despite his superior intellectual ability. Although he consciously stated his desire for success and that he did not know why he was such a procrastinator, his passive-aggressive behavior effectively defeated his parents and rendered them powerless.

Schizoid fantasy is a mechanism in which there is a denial and retreat from problems in the external world. It serves to provide partial gratification of unmet needs for interpersonal relationships or to bolster self-esteem. A clinical illustration is that of an awkward adolescent boy who developed an extensive fantasy world in which he was a soldier-of-fortune who experienced numerous adventures and sexual conquests. If these fantasies had been communicated to someone else as if they were true, then they would be called pseudologia fantastica.

Dissociation is the mechanism by which one compartmentalizes ideas, memories, or experiences that may elicit intolerable feelings, moving them out of conscious awareness. For example, a rape victim has only vague memories of the assault on her. The specific details have been recorded in her memory and may be available through hypnosis or sodium Amytal interviews, but they are not readily accessible by conscious intent. Dissociation is closely related to psychiatric disorders such as multiple personality disorder (dissociative identity disorder) and fugue states. It has been suggested that memories of childhood traumas (such as sexual abuse) may be dissociated, leading to future psychiatric disorders.

David Spiegel, professor of psychiatry at Stanford University, has made dissociation one of his major research interests. He has found that dissociative phenomena occur frequently in healthy people after they experience a traumatic event. For example, he and his colleagues (Freinkel et al. 1994) found that seasoned media reporters who witnessed an execution were prone to dissociative periods in the weeks following the event.

Displacement describes the process of moving one's fears and concerns from a highly conflictive and anxiety-provoking situation to one that is more controllable. For example, a woman dying of lung cancer became preoccupied with her constipation rather than focusing on symptoms that reflected her respiratory failure. A man who had a conflictive and suffocating relationship with his intrusive and controlling mother found it easier to believe, and explain to others, that he could not visit her in her high-rise condominium because his claustrophobia prevented him from using elevators.

Intellectualization, isolation, and *rationalization* are terms used to describe closely related and often interlocking ego mechanisms. Individuals are aware of the external facts of a situation but isolate emotion and often attempt to provide reasons to explain their behavior. An easily recognized example of intellectualization and isolation is the experience of a freshman medical student in a course on gross anatomy. At the beginning of the course, the student has considerable anxiety and dread about how to relate to the cadaver, which is perceived as a "dead person"; by the end of the course, any feelings of a humanistic nature toward the cadaver have been isolated. Dissection of the cadaver has approximately the same emotional impact as a chemistry experiment.

A dramatic lesson in an extreme use of intellectualization, rationalization, and isolation is the behavior of physicians in Nazi Germany (Lifton 1982; Trepman 1988). These doctors, highly cultured and ostensibly devoted to the preservation of human life, conducted unethical and often brutal experiments with Jewish subjects. They also frequently played major roles in the administration and functions of the death camps. Dr. Edward Wirths, chief physician at Auschwitz, carried out lethal and mutilating experiments and worked as a camp physician, deciding who should be gassed. Yet Wirths was described by those who knew him as a husband with close family ties, a loving father, and a husband who wrote passionate love letters to his wife. There appeared to be two Dr. Wirths—one was a war criminal, and the other was a loving father and husband. The only explanation, short of psychosis, is that Dr. Wirths kept the two sides separate from each other. He isolated his emotional responses to his "work" as a Nazi doctor, rationalizing his behavior as duty to his country. What incredible self-deception! Wirths eventually committed suicide but only after the Allied liberation of Auschwitz (Lifton 1986).

Reaction formation describes feelings or behaviors that are opposite to an unacceptable impulse, wish, or fear. For example, the superficially sweet demeanor of the southern belle may disguise—from others and herself—underlying anger and resentment. An unconscious fear of disease and death may motivate someone into studying and practicing medicine, and a person who is fearful of heights may become a sky diver.

Repression refers to the process of blocking from consciousness those ideas or feelings that provoke anxiety or are painful to experience. Repression may include lapses of memory or the failure to acknowledge one's feelings. It is not uncommon in psychotherapy for patients to exhibit all of the behavioral and psychological features of anger while denying that they have feelings of anger (Ford and Long 1977).

Some ego-defense mechanisms have proven to be more adaptive than others.

Altruism describes a process in which one receives vicarious pleasure by providing service to others. A nurse caring for others may vicariously receive some gratification of her own dependency wishes. A well-to-do childless couple made substantial contributions every Christmas to various agencies that provided gifts to needy children. In addition, each Christmas morning they knocked on the doors and gave inexpensive, but carefully chosen, gifts to each child on the block on which they lived. These genuinely kind people delighted in being addressed as "Uncle Tom" and "Aunt Mary" by the neighborhood children. The process of altruism defends against the awareness of one's own wishes for nurturance through vicariously receiving pleasure by providing for the needs of others.

Anticipation is realistic planning for future intrapsychic discomfort; it is also the capacity to achieve some pleasure from delayed gratification. A psychologically healthy family with a terminally ill member does some anticipatory mourning, so that the inevitable loss does not come as a shock and overwhelm the family's capacity to cope. A medical or law student may sacrifice many hours of pleasure in order to study, while achieving some satisfaction in knowing that the reward for such self-sacrifice will be gratifying.

Sublimation is the process by which instinctual drives are attenuated by a socially accepted means. The high energy and aggression characteristic of male adolescents can be channeled into socially accepted athletic endeavors. Artistic works can be a creative way of expressing one's emotions.

Suppression differs from repression in that one consciously or subconsciously excludes thoughts or feelings from the conscious but retrieves the memories and deals with them at the appropriate time. It is an efficient method to set aside mental tasks without ignoring them.

Humor is the ability to be playful and to laugh at oneself. It differs from wit, which may be a sadistic attack on another person. The person who has learned to use humor can accept personal failings ("nobody is perfect") without a devastating loss of self-esteem. Humor helps to maintain relationships with others, and thus the individual benefits from continuing support from the social system.

Relation of Ego-Defense Mechanisms to Self-Deception

Vaillant (1971) proposed a theoretical hierarchy of the maturity level of various ego-defense mechanisms (Table 2–3). He used a long-term prospective study of men to evaluate the specific defense mechanisms used by individuals and then correlated the use of different defense mechanisms with the quality of the man's adjustment to life. Individuals with the best life adjustment scores characteristically used a variety of different defenses, predominantly those that were considered mature or neurotic. Individuals with "good" or "fair" life adjustment scores were more likely to use neurotic or immature defenses. Vaillant's initial work was later confirmed by the use of a different group of subjects and alternative measurement techniques (Vaillant et al. 1986).

Support for the concept of a hierarchy of ego mechanisms has also been generated by Cramer (1987), who identified a shift from

---

Table 2–3.   Ego-defense mechanisms

Level 1: Narcissistic
  Denial
  Delusional projection
  Distortion

Level 2: Immature
  Projection
  Acting out
  Hypochondriasis
  Passive-aggressive behavior
  Schizoid fantasy

Level 3: Neurotic
  Dissociation
  Displacement
  Intellectualization
  Isolation
  Rationalization
  Reaction formation
  Repression

Level 4: Mature
  Altruism
  Anticipation
  Sublimation
  Suppression
  Humor

Source.   Adapted from Vaillant GE: "Theoretical Hierarchy of Adaptive Ego Mechanisms." *Archives of General Psychiatry* 24:107–118, 1971.

denial to more mature ego mechanisms as children grow older and develop. Ford and Spaulding (1973) found that the capacity to adjust to the severe stressors of being held hostage was related to both the maturity and the flexibility of the individual's defensive structure. Vaillant and Vaillant (1990) determined that an important predictor for mental health in later life was the maturity of the defenses as identified before age 50.

In reviewing ego-defense mechanisms, it is notable that the level of maturity (as specified by Vaillant) appears highly correlated with the degree of self-deception. With level-one defenses (narcissistic), reality is distorted or disavowed. Self-deception at this level is so great that it interferes with reality testing. With level-two defenses (immature), the individual remains largely unaware of thoughts and feelings that are acted on with maladaptive behavior or that are disavowed and projected to another individual. With level-three defenses (neurotic), self-deception is largely manifested by the compartmentalization of mental activity. There is a considerable increase in one's awareness, ideas, and emotions, but the ambivalence of a conflictive issue may be kept out of consciousness by "splitting." Active self-deception is most readily identified at this level. Self-deception also occurs with defense mechanisms at level four (mature), but it is under more conscious control and is more adaptive. The mature defenses also tend to promote and improve relationships with others.

To some degree, self-deception is necessary for good mental health. This provocative idea will be further explored in Chapter 13, in which the relation of self-deception to the maintenance of self-esteem is explored. However, deceiving oneself to the extent that basic reality testing is impaired is clearly detrimental.

Summary

The English language has a rich variety of words to describe the phenomenon of lying. Technically, one may deceive even while telling the truth and lie without deceiving. Lies may be classified by a variety of categorizations, including the degree of malignancy or to whom the lie is told.

Deceit is not produced by words alone. In fact, nonverbal communication can be remarkably deceptive, and the ability to control one's nonverbal behavior is essential to becoming a skilled liar.

We deceive ourselves as well as others; to a large extent such self-deception is mediated through ego-defense mechanisms. A high level of self-deception is characteristic of the more primitive and immature defense mechanisms, but the self-deception associated with mature ego-defense mechanisms appears to be highly adaptive.

Chapter 3

The Biology of Deceit

A male [baboon], one who does not willingly share,
caught an antelope. The female edged up to him and
groomed him until he lulled under her attentions. She
then snatched the antelope carcass and ran.

—Lewin 1987

Do animals lie? What are the data to indicate that deceit exists in the animal kingdom in species other than *Homo sapiens*? The investigation of animal behaviors (the sciences of ethology and sociobiology) has been a valuable tool for understanding the role of instinct across different species. Such investigations will eventually allow us to better comprehend the functions of basic brain mechanisms that underlie human behaviors. Thus, the study of deceit in animals may have implications for determining certain underlying factors that influence different types of deceit, both verbal and nonverbal, in humans.

Deceit in Lower Species

If one considers camouflage a form of deception, then deceit is certainly the rule of thumb in the animal kingdom (Wile 1942). In a world of predators, it is important that an animal makes itself inconspicuous so it is not noticed and devoured. Another strategy is to make itself appear so fearsome that potential predators will leave it alone. Similarly, the predator often has coloring and behaviors that disguise its presence or intentions, thus increasing its success in stalking prey. Survival for both predator and prey is continuously at stake: the ability to send false information improves the chances of living another day.

According to the theory of evolution, characteristics that increase reproductive rates will be differentially selected. Reproductive success is obviously influenced by the mere fact of survival to and through reproductive age. Differential reproduction is also influenced by factors that promote both the frequency and appropriate timing of mating, as well as the capability of caring for young. Thus, features of an individual that increase opportunities for sexual behavior are likely to be reflected in natural selection. The following examples illustrate how various forms of "deceit" in lower species may promote basic survival and opportunities for mating.

Many forms of deception in animals are passive in nature and do not require behavior per se. An animal's coloring may blend into the background so that the creature is not easily seen. Some animals have coats that shed and grow again with different colorations to match the foliage of the season. Other animals have reflexive changes that, when threatened, make them appear more formidable; for example, the piloerection (the bristling of fur) of canines makes them seem larger and more fearsome. Similarly, the blowfish inflates and extends its spiny fins when a potential predator is near.

Many species of birds behave in ways to distract or divert predators in order to protect their eggs or young. Sordahl (1986) systematically studied two species of birds (the American avocet and the black-necked stilt), watching behaviors that appear to deceive certain predators. These birds "dive-bomb" toward the predator while making a sound that increases in frequency as the bird approaches the target. This increased pitch enhances the Doppler effect, thereby increasing the target's perception of the bird's speed (and presumably the capacity to frighten the predator away from the eggs or young birds). Interestingly, these birds actually have soft bills and little ability to inflict injury to a predator.

Other behaviors include a "crouch-run" display that conveys a sense of furtiveness, a wing display that indicates injury, and a false incubation display (behaving as if the birds studied by Sordahl were incubating eggs and brooding the young). Each of these behaviors occurs with high frequency at the time of incubation and brooding, although the frequency of specific behaviors tends to change with different phases of incubation or with the type of risk from a predator. Sordahl reported that these behaviors cause predators to leave or to be diverted from the true position of the eggs or fledglings.

The communication of fireflies by their flashes is so fraught with deceit that Lloyd (1986) called it "deception as a way of life" (p. 124). The fireflies' flashes serve as sexual communication. For example, the male *Photinus pyralis* emits a half-second flash about every 6 seconds while flying in a J-shaped swoop over shrubs or clumps of grass where a female is likely to be perched. A responsive female will wait 2 seconds after the male's flash and then emit her own half-second flash. The sequence may be repeated a dozen or more times before the male finally reaches and mounts the female. However, because a female immediately begins laying eggs after mating (and is thus "out of circulation"), there is a surplus of males.

This surplus of males is used to the advantage of another firefly of the genus *Photuris*. The female *Photuris* mimics the response signals of the female *Photinus pyralis* to attract the male of that genus and then eats him! Adding yet another twist to this deceptive pattern, the male *Photuris*, when flying low, may mimic the signal of the male *Photinus* to find *Photuris* females with which to mate.

Lloyd described other quirks of firefly behavior, including that sometimes a mimic may mimic a mimic! He concluded that "where there are eggs to be fertilized and nurtured, deception is sure to make an appearance" (p. 126). One cannot help but conclude that this tongue-in-cheek observation is applicable to many species, including *Homo sapiens*.

Alarm calls are vocal warnings that one individual of a species of bird may emit to warn that a predator is near. Such warnings, for example, may cause a mixed-species flock of birds to scatter. Munn (1986) described the use of deceptive alarm calls by several species of "sentinels." These birds warn of the approach of predator hawks, and the flock takes protective action. However, the alarm may be used deceptively to the sentinel's advantage. For example, if the flock has flushed a number of arthropods, a false signal that scatters the flock then gives the deceiver an advantage in catching the prey. These false alarms occur more frequently when the perpetrators are feeding fledglings, suggesting that the trick is reserved for a time when there is a greater need for extra food.

The preceding descriptions suggest that deceptive behaviors in some lower species have their origins in instinct or learned behavior. One would not ascribe human motivations to them. It has been proposed that without a sense of self and differentiation from others, it would be impossible to consciously discern the motivations of another individual (e.g., the conscious intent to induce a false belief in another individual). Following this reasoning, the presence of consciously determined deception is presumed evidence of a sense of self (Premack 1988; Wimmer et al. 1985).

Thus, deception experiments in animals and children have often had the common goal of searching for developmental evidence of the capacity to see others as separate: at what points along the evolutionary pathways do animals develop sufficient neurological capability for conscious or humanlike deception? Some might argue that all animals are innocent and only humans are capable of motivated dishonesty. However, observations of the more intelligent animal species suggest, at the risk of anthropomorphic interpretation, that the behaviors seem strikingly humanlike. Certainly the vignette described at the beginning of this chapter suggests consciously motivated and planned deceptive behavior. Other behaviors with a quality of purposefulness have also been described in higher primates and elephants.

Deceit in Elephants and Primates

From her observations of elephants at the Washington Park Zoo (Portland, Oregon), Morris (1986) concluded that elephants can recognize the correlation between their own behavior and others' responses. This knowledge can be used in a manipulative manner. For example, to activate the shower at the zoo, one elephant must pull a chain for another elephant's benefit. Morris observed that a certain elephant, Pet, appeared to thwart potentially antagonistic encounters with her rival, Hanako, by pulling the chain for her. However, on several occasions, Pet would act as if she were about to pull the chain and then stop when Hanako moved toward the sprayer. This feigned shower initiation by Pet (which from an anthropomorphic perspective seems markedly passive-aggressive) eventually resulted in Hanako attacking Pet.

Frans deWaal (1986, 1988) studied chimpanzees at the primate facility of the Arnhem Zoo (in The Netherlands). He concluded that "deception seems to permeate all aspects of the chimpanzees' social life, and chimpanzees' skills in deceit are a match for human lie-detecting abilities" (deWaal 1986, p. 240). The chimpanzees' ability to deceive humans was exhibited in one characteristic female behavior described as the "lure." One female chimpanzee, Jimi, was known for her trick of offering a blade of straw to a stranger while maintaining a poker face. Just as the person (the victim) would take the "gift," Jimi would quickly grab the person with her other hand. Similar luring behaviors of female apes have been reported by others.

An observed male behavior was illustrated by Nikkie, a chimpanzee known for his habit of throwing well-aimed heavy objects. He aggressively pursued a female, who was able to avoid him by using a tree trunk as cover. However, as she moved to the right, Nikkie threw a brick and then quickly turned to the left so he could capture her as she jumped back to the left to avoid the missile. The high degree of coordination of this maneuver left little doubt in the observers that it was intentional and that Nikkie was able to anticipate his victim's reaction. Such anticipation is a critical component of successful deception.

Another behavior observed in chimpanzees seems to imply aspects of self-deception. After a negative experience (e.g., being defeated in a power struggle with another chimpanzee), a chimpanzee may turn his attention to something unimportant, such as careful examination of his fingernails, to hide what appears to be embarrassment. Face-saving tactics have also been noted among other primates, and deWaal (1986) commented that it is tempting to regard these behaviors as collective lies because one party deceives and the other acts as if it has been deceived. For example, if a dominant monkey threatens a subordinate one, the subordinate monkey may act as if the signal was never received by not looking in the direction of the dominant monkey. The dominant monkey may then "let things go," because if no "orders" were received, then the lack of a response cannot be regarded as a challenge. Thus, one monkey pretends not to receive the message, and the other monkey agrees to the deception.

The behaviors and politics of primates, especially the great apes, seem strikingly human. Is it because we project human motivations into our observations, or is it because many human behaviors have evolved from common origins? Ethologists (scientists who study animal behavior) have proposed that many human behaviors are derived from instinctual patterns that evolved in lower species. One important area to investigate is the evolution of social behavior (Trivers 1985).

Reciprocal Altruism and Deceit

If deception and the detection of deception are effective survival strategies for an individual, there should be natural selection for increasingly better methods of deceit and its detection. These strategies for the individual appear to be in contrast to the evolution of social relationships of higher species and humans that are characterized by shared communications, trust, and altruistic behaviors. Altruism, as used here, is defined as behavior that benefits another organism (not closely related) but is apparently detrimental to the organism performing the behavior. Robert Trivers (1971), in a classic paper in theoretical biology, addressed this apparent contradiction in his proposal of the concept of reciprocal altruism. Associated with the concept are Trivers' speculations about how and why the human brain has evolved.

Reciprocal altruism can be viewed as a form of symbiosis, with each party helping the other parties while helping itself. An immediate payoff (reciprocation) is not needed if the potential for long-term benefit exists. Trivers suggested that several conditions must be met for such reciprocity to exist. These conditions include a long life span, low dispersal rates, individual recognition, and a degree of mutual dependence. These factors increase the probability of multiple encounters with the same network of individuals. Trivers cited the cleaning behaviors of marine life and warning calls of birds as examples of reciprocal altruism that occur in lower species when the aforementioned conditions are present.

Human reciprocal altruism probably evolved during the Pleistocene epoch, when the hominid species would have met the conditions listed above for reciprocal altruism.

A partial list of altruistic behaviors includes helping others in times of danger, sharing food, assisting the sick and wounded, and—very important for the purpose of this treatise—sharing knowledge. To benefit the individual engaging in these acts of altruism, which by definition provide immediate benefit to another individual, the acts must be repaid at some future time.

On the surface, cheating—that is, taking without giving—benefits the one who cheats. One strategy is to learn to be a subtle cheater, repaying with less than what was received. However, when individuals become known as cheaters, resentment will probably cause others to reduce their assistance to those individuals. Thus, the social group (other members of the species) develops methods to control cheaters. For example, members of a group may take an aggressive moralistic action toward cheaters by socializing them, through fear or exclusion, into reciprocal altruistic behavior. In severe situations, cheaters may be killed or excluded from the social group.

The rehabilitation of a cheater involves remorse and reparative altruism to the social group. Displays of contrition may then allow the individual to again receive altruistic acts from the social network. This condition allows a new type of deceit: sham guilt. The subtle cheater may pretend to be contrite in order to gain rewards, while continuing to cheat. This behavior is well recognized in persons who treat alcoholic patients. The extreme remorsefulness shown by alcoholic individuals is frequently not followed by changes in behavior (see Chapter 7).

The existence of sham guilt exerts a new pressure on individuals to make determinations about guilt and remorseful behavior. Is a remorseful expression genuine, or is it merely another form of deceit? The altruist must ensure that there is, in fact, reciprocity; after all, no one wants to be a "sucker." On the other hand, sham moralistic aggression may exist as another form of cheating; that is, one can impute cheating motives to another to hide one's own cheating.

Trivers suggested that this complex system, in which there are selective advantages for both the effective cheater and those individuals who are able to detect cheating, has produced selective evolutionary pressure for cognitive and psychological powers. That is, there has been ever-increasing competition for effective deception and its detection. He postulated that this growing interplay of deceit and its detection may have contributed to the large increase in brain size during the later stages of human evolution. Trivers (1988) also suggested that self-deception may have evolved as a mechanism to facilitate "other-deception." People lie more effectively if they "believe" what they are saying.

Trivers' concept of reciprocal altruism provides a theoretical model for use in studying the biological components of deceit in humans, the role of deceit in social interchange, and the origins of moral systems.

Neurological Substrates of Deceit

Any biological consideration of factors related to deceit must examine the brain and its functions. Certain instinctive brain mechanisms account for deceitful behaviors in lower species, and it is not unreasonable to assume that some fundamental remnant of these processes persists in humans.

In the past, much of what was known about the localization of brain function came from clinical studies of individuals who had experienced a loss of brain matter after a stroke or trauma. Assessment of the specific damage to the brain would be delayed until a postmortem examination could be completed. Yet, it was learned, for example, that tissue damage to the motor cortex was associated with paralysis in a fairly specific manner and that damage to the dominant temporal cortex was associated with speech impairment.

It is now possible to use technology to gain a much more accurate picture of the living brain (Andreasen 1989). Computed tomography (CT) and magnetic resonance imaging (MRI) create computer-generated pictures of cross-sections of living brain tissue, providing details of cortical and subcortical structures of white and gray matter. Furthermore, brain metabolic activity can be displayed by the use of positron-emission tomography (PET) or single photon emission computed tomography (SPECT). Thus, pictures of the living brain can be created that reflect different psychological or physiological states. The electroencephalogram (EEG), long used in clinical neurology, is limited to monitoring the electrical activity of the brain's surface. However, recent improvements in the EEG, using computerized methods for displaying electrical activity, have made it possible to provide visual pictures of brain electrical activity. This process is called brain electrical activity mapping (BEAM). Some of these new technologies have already been used to study neurological aspects of deceit, and they will become increasingly common investigational tools during the coming decade.

In consideration of the possible roles of neurological substrates of deceit, I briefly review the functions of the prefrontal lobes and the hemispheric structure of the brain in human behavior. The neurological mechanisms that are related to confabulation may cast some light on our understanding of lying and self-deception.

Prefrontal Lobes in Human Behavior

The prefrontal lobes are the most recently evolved structures of the human brain. They are the site of interconnections and feedback loops among the major sensory and motor systems. The prefrontal cortex receives information from all sources—conscious and unconscious, internal and external—and integrates all components of behavior (Lezak 1983).

Damage to the prefrontal lobes does not always cause obvious deficits in cognitive or motor functioning. Intelligence, as measured by IQ testing, for example, may be minimally affected even by relatively severe tissue loss (Lezak 1983). For this reason, the term *silent lesion* has been used to describe pathological changes in the prefrontal lobes. However, well-established syndromes of behavioral changes occur with prefrontal-lobe damage. Most of these are characterized by impaired social judgment.

Blumer and Benson (1975) described the pseudopsychopathic personality syndrome that can follow injury to the orbital frontal lobe or to neural pathways crossing that part of the brain. Individuals with this syndrome are characterized by lack of tact and normal restraint; they may be coarse, irritable, fractious, hyperkinetic, or promiscuous. They usually lack social graces and sensitivity for others, yet are guileless in their acknowledgment of their behaviors. For example, they may engage in inappropriate sexual talk, show little embarrassment about bathroom functions, or have disregard for traffic laws. However, unlike persons with a true sociopathic personality, they generally make little effort to deny responsibility for their behaviors. They may become angry in an emotionally unstable manner, but they do not tend to bear grudges.

Another type of frontal-lobe syndrome is associated with injury to the convexity of the prefrontal lobes and certain subcortical centers, particularly the basal ganglia, thalamus, and their connections (Blumer and Benson 1975). These persons often have a pseudodepressive syndrome marked by slowness, apathy, and a loss of initiative. These changes were noted in the patients who had undergone early massive prefrontal lobotomies for psychiatric illnesses. The pseudopsychopathic and pseudodepressive syndromes rarely appear in their pure forms; usually some mixture of the two is found.

"Split Brain"

Can one part of the brain deceive another part? Research in brain function over the past several decades has established that the two hemispheres of the brain have different functions and can at times operate somewhat independently of each other. These findings are important to our understanding of deceit because they imply that a neurological substrate may cause the apparent contradiction in the term *self-deception.*

Most people have a dominant hemisphere of the brain (usually the left side in right-handed persons) and a nondominant hemisphere. Each hemisphere controls the motor activities of the other side of the body. The dominant side is specialized and mediates functions of language, speech, and logic. The nondominant side is involved in processing information related to music and spatial functions, such as recognizing faces. The two hemispheres communicate with each other through the corpus callosum and, to a lesser degree, through the anterior commissure.

In an effort to treat intractable epilepsy, Dr. Joseph Bogen (1985), a neurosurgeon in southern California, has performed cerebral commissurotomies (i.e., severance of the corpus callosum in a neurosurgical procedure), a procedure that is usually effective in controlling some types of epilepsy. As a result of these operations, Dr. Bogen's patients have "split brains." After surgical recovery, the neurological and psychological states of his patients have been carefully investigated.

One neurological finding is a specific form of aphasia or apraxia in which postcommissurotomy patients cannot follow verbal commands to move parts of the left sides of their bodies. The left side of the body is not paralyzed, and the person can move it if the movement is modeled by another person. Also, they cannot recognize written words presented only to their nondominant visual fields. Surprisingly, these split-brain patients, although unable to identify a common song immediately, can eventually call out the title after humming along with the tune (Gazzaniga et al. 1975). The separation of the "two brains" was illustrated by one patient who was seen buttoning his shirt with one hand, while the other hand followed along behind it undoing the buttons. Truly, the right hand did not know what the left hand was doing!

Klaus Hoppe, a psychoanalyst who worked with Dr. Bogen, carefully evaluated these split-brain patients. He found that they exhibited an impoverishment of dreams, fantasies, and symbol systems (Hoppe 1977; Hoppe and Bogen 1977). He observed that these findings were remarkably similar to alexithymic persons who have been identified as having psychosomatic illnesses. Alexithymia means "without words for mood" and describes people who are unable to verbally communicate their emotional states. One alexithymic patient whom I treated in group therapy became agitated, turned red, stood up, and scowled. When asked why he was angry, he appeared perplexed and denied that he was upset (Ford and Long 1977). Features commonly associated with alexithymia include a lack of psychological mindedness (i.e., the capacity to relate emotions to behavior), an impoverished fantasy life, and an inability to remember dreams.

Hoppe proposed that persons with alexithymia may have a "functional commissurotomy." Despite anatomically intact nerve tracts, the transfer of information from one side of their brains to the other is inhibited. Certainly, these alexithymic patients are out of contact (self-deceived?) with their emotional states. This understanding of the bilateral brain provides one possibility about how self-deception can occur.

Neurological Syndromes Related to Deceit

The neurological syndromes of confabulation and reduplicative paramnesia appear to be related to pseudologia fantastica. I review these syndromes in conjunction with those neuropsychological findings that have been associated with pseudologia fantastica.

Confabulation

Stuss and colleagues (1978) described confabulation as the production of erroneous and fabricated verbal material caused by an inability to be self-critical rather than a deliberate effort to mislead. Confabulation has traditionally been associated with Wernicke-Korsakoff syndrome. This neurological disorder is caused by a thiamine deficiency and is characterized by dysfunction of midbrain structures that control memory and other functions, such as eye movements (Victor et al. 1971). In its more common form, termed *provoked confabulation* by Kopelman (1987a), it is a transient, limited, and unspectacular response to a direct question (Berlyne 1972). The provoked response may be quite nonsensical, but the patient has little awareness of any absurdity. Confabulation is assumed to be an effort to fill memory gaps, and although it may be a prominent symptom in patients who have memory deficits (e.g., Wernicke-Korsakoff syndrome or Alzheimer's disease), it is very similar to the ways in which healthy persons compensate for memory gaps. This has been demonstrated in an experimental study using a medication (scopolamine) to impair anterograde (short-term) memory in healthy subjects (Kopelman 1987b).

Spontaneous confabulation is a less common and more psycho-pathological phenomenon. Patients with this condition impulsively provide more spectacular and spontaneous false information. They do not merely respond to a question with an inaccurate answer as in provoked confabulation; rather, they embellish their answers in an attempt to impress the audience. Even when the amnesia is mild, the confabulation can be striking. For example, one patient studied by Stuss and colleagues (1978) fabricated a story of sustaining a head injury while trying to rescue one of his children during a drowning accident.

Early etiological concepts of confabulation emphasized memory deficit in conjunction with premorbid personality traits (those that were present before the brain damage) or suggestibility (Berlyne 1972). It has also been suggested that the major difficulty for these patients is the ability to organize the context of their memories. In other words, memories from the past may be confused with memories of the present (Victor et al. 1971). Furthermore, Weinstein (1971) described the content of confabulations as metaphorical representations of current problems. For example, he described a military officer whose intellectual deficits following a head injury had disqualified him from further service; the officer told a story about having been engaged in counterintelligence activities.

Longitudinal evaluations of confabulation indicate that confabulation is not related to either the extent of memory loss or suggestibility (Mercer et al. 1977). Mercer and colleagues attributed confabulation to the coincidence of four factors: 1) the belief that a response is required, 2) an absence of a memory for the answer, 3) the availability of an overlearned and affectively significant response, and 4) a defective ability to monitor and self-correct for inaccurate responses. It must also be emphasized that confabulation is not an all-or-nothing phenomenon. A patient may at times admit to not knowing the answer and at other times confabulate. Sometimes the patient may recognize a response as inaccurate and make an effort to correct it.

The major neurophysiological issue in confabulation does not appear to be memory deficit itself but the manner in which the patient manages the memory deficit. Several investigators have emphasized that spontaneous confabulation requires a memory deficit in conjunction with frontal-lobe dysfunction (Kapur and Coughlan

1980; Kopelman 1987a; Mayes et al. 1985; Stuss et al. 1978). It has been suggested that the frontal lobes provide a context for memories, integrating current environmental cues with past experiences. The frontal lobes also provide a self-correcting mechanism to ensure the accuracy of verbal responses. When the neurological system is dysfunctional, verbal responses can be impulsive, and—because of associated memories—neutral material may be presented in an emotionally charged manner.

Joseph (1986) proposed that the speech area of the dominant hemisphere may occasionally be unable to access and assimilate relevant information. At those times, the individual substitutes other material, resulting in confabulation. If the speech area is isolated from other areas of the brain on which it depends for judgment, moral values, and analysis, it cannot recognize the absurdity of what the individual is saying. Joseph suggests that this phenomenon may occur in self-deception because of functional, rather than anatomical, disconnections. Thus, "gap filling" may provide an explanation for behaviors or impulses that seem reasonable, innocuous, and accurate but that are erroneous.

Reduplicative Paramnesia

Reduplicative paramnesia, a neurological syndrome following brain injury, is similar to confabulation in many respects (Benson et al. 1976). Patients with this syndrome demonstrate a persistent relocation of their orientation to place, despite their apparent recovery of memory functions to near-normal levels. For example, one man with reduplicative paramnesia repeatedly insisted that he was in another city, despite frequent efforts of family and physicians to correct his misperceptions. His cognitive abilities were apparently intact, and he had a Wechsler Adult Intelligence Scale (WAIS) IQ of 114.[1] The verbal IQ was 127, but his performance IQ

---

[1]Intelligence tests are scored in a manner that allows a comparison with the performance of an average person. A score of 100 is defined as average, and each 10 points or below represent 1 standard deviation from the average. Only about 5% of the population score as high as 120 for either the WAIS IQ Scale or the Wechsler Memory Scale.

was 97; the Wechsler Memory Scale at this time was 137, well into the superior range. Benson and colleagues indicated that each of their patients with reduplicative paramnesia had evidence of significant damage to the frontal lobes and disproportionate damage to the nondominant hemisphere of the brain, which controls the functions of visual and spatial orientation. They suggested that significant right-hemispheric pathology may be a necessary precondition for reduplicative paramnesia. They further suggested that decreased frontal-lobe function might be the source of a prolonged inability to correct geographical disorientation, even in the face of otherwise adequate memory functions.

Relation of Neurological Dysfunction to Deceit

Some forms of deceit that have been described as pathological lying may have a neurological basis.

Pseudologia Fantastica

Pseudologia fantastica is a dramatic form of pathological lying (see Chapters 2 and 7) that consists of grandiose stories with a matrix of truth and fiction (King and Ford 1988). In some respects, this syndrome resembles spontaneous confabulation (or "fantastic confabulation"), except no memory disturbance is apparent. When vigorously confronted, the pseudologue can acknowledge the fabrications as falsehoods. Pseudologia fantastica may occur as a separate phenomenon or as part of other psychiatric syndromes, such as factitious disorder or imposture. It is a predominant feature of the Munchausen syndrome, an extreme manifestation of factitious disorder. Other features of pseudologia fantastica are discussed in Chapters 7 and 8; this discussion focuses on neurological aspects.

In their extensive review, King and Ford (1988) noted that 40% of recorded cases of pseudologia fantastica occurred in patients with a history of some brain abnormality, primarily epilepsy, abnormal EEG, head trauma, or central nervous system infection. Among the limited number of patients for whom intelligence testing had been reported, a majority showed verbal abilities (dominant-hemispheric functions) that were significantly better than performance abilities (nondominant-hemispheric functions). This finding is similar to the discrepancy between verbal and performance IQ reported in patients with confabulation (Berlyne 1972; Stuss et al. 1978).

Pancratz and Lezak (1987) found that of the 25 Munchausen syndrome patients they assessed, about one-third had serious brain dysfunction. They reported specific neuropsychological results for 5 patients who had startling variance among their test scores. These patients were all verbal, facile with medical terminology, and had an impressive fund of knowledge. Yet each had deficits of judgment, conceptual organization, and management of complex information. Pancratz and Lezak acknowledged that the neuropsychological deficits may have been the result, rather than the cause, of the patients' behavior (e.g., having sought and received multiple surgical operations and the effects of drug abuse). Nevertheless, it was proposed that Munchausen syndrome could serve as a psychodynamic solution to critical problems with which the patient was trying to cope, including brain dysfunction. They noted that the pseudologia was similar to the product of the illogical reasoning and lack of verbal inhibition found in confabulation patients with nondominant-hemispheric and frontal-lobe dysfunction, as previously described by Weinstein (1971).

A case report of a patient with compulsive lying also points to frontal-lobe dysfunction as a potential contributing etiological factor (Modell et al. 1992). This 35-year-old man's propensity to lie began when he was about age 25 years. It involved issues as trivial as where he put the tissue box and serious matters such as falsely claiming to have completed work assignments. He stated that he could not recognize his falsehoods until "I hear the words slipping out of my mouth." Psychiatric consultation was precipitated by his wife's threat of divorce. On evaluation, he did not meet diagnostic criteria for any psychiatric or personality disorder, except for adjustment problems. However, neuropsychological testing demonstrated evidence of mild tactile and sensory perceptual difficulty on the left side of the body, upper-right extremity weakness, and mild short-term memory impairment. A CT scan of the head, gadolinium-enhanced MRI scan of the head, and sleep-deprived EEG were all normal. However, two SPECT scans of the head that were performed 2 weeks apart revealed abnormally low activity in the right hemithalamus (nondominant), an area of the brain responsible for the integration of sensory stimuli, and the right inferior frontal cortex, an area of the brain that has multiple inputs from other parts of the brain and integrates these stimuli into appropriate social responses. The authors hypothesized that his dysfunction may have reduced internal feedback, causing the tendency to lie without recognizing the veracity of his speech until after he heard it spoken.

The above data, although tentative, suggest the importance of both frontal-lobe and nondominant-hemispheric function in the self-regulation of accuracy of verbal productions. Similarities between confabulation and pseudologia fantastica are striking, and differences may be largely quantitative, reflecting the degree of impaired memory function.

Cognitive Style

The descriptions above of mild confabulation—characterized by impulsive, affective statements—resemble the hysterical cognitive style (see Chapter 6). To my knowledge, the issue of cognitive style has not been specifically investigated using neuropsychological techniques. However, patients with "hysteria" (somatization disorder) have been evaluated by Flor-Henry and associates (1981). They found dominant-hemispheric dysfunction with some nondominant impairment in these patients. Interestingly, cluster analysis (a type of statistical evaluation) of their test results showed that patients with somatization disorder were more similar to schizophrenic patients than they were to depressed patients. Schizophrenia is now believed to be closely related to reduced function of the prefrontal lobes.

Sociopathy and hysteria share a similar cognitive style (impulsive and shaped by emotion) and have been linked in family studies. Women with hysteria (somatization disorder) have more male relatives with sociopathy than would be expected by chance (Arkonac and Guze 1963), and it has been suggested that the two disorders are closely related, with symptomatic expression being determined by gender (Guze et al. 1971). Of importance in this regard is the study of Gorenstein (1982), who found that persons with sociopathic personality disorder exhibited similar performance patterns on neuropsychological tests as did patients with frontal-lobe lesions.

More recent research further supports the suggestion that certain personality characteristics—including how information is processed—are influenced by cognitive dysfunction. Burgess (1992) used neuropsychological tests to study patients in the "dramatic cluster" (Cluster B) of personality disorders. This cluster includes the histrionic, narcissistic, borderline, and antisocial personality disorders (these personality disorders are discussed in detail in Chapter 6). Burgess found that these patients have significant deficiencies in the neurocognitive functions of attention, memory, language, abstraction, and behavior planning and sequencing. O'Leary and colleagues (1991) used neuropsychological tests to study persons with borderline personality disorder. These patients scored poorly on tests requiring uncued recall of complex, recently learned material. The investigators concluded that the person with borderline personality disorder may have difficulties separating essential from extraneous visual information and retrieving complex material from memory.

As noted above, because of many shared similarities, certain personality disorders are placed together as Cluster B in DSM-IV (American Psychiatric Association 1994). Of note, one characteristic of all the Cluster B personality disorders is the propensity for lying. The above findings, although preliminary and tentative, suggest that underlying neurocognitive dysfunction may be associated with certain types of personality disorders and that this dysfunction may play a role in the frequent use of lying as a coping mechanism. One extension of this line of thought is derived from Trivers' hypothesis about the evolution of the human brain. Lying associated with brain dysfunction is likely to be crude rather than subtle; that crudeness is probably due to a lower level of social awareness of the impact of the deceit. This trait is characteristic of many persons who have Cluster B personality disorders. One must keep in mind, however, that an associated finding is not the same as a cause. Subtle cognitive impairment might arise from consequences of the personality disorder (such as substance abuse) rather than be a cause of the disorder.

In many respects, the obsessive-compulsive cognitive style (see Chapter 6) is the converse of the hysterical style. Neural imaging studies of patients who have obsessive-compulsive disorder have shown increased activity in the orbital portions of the frontal lobe (Nordahl et al. 1989; Swedo et al. 1989).

Hereditary Influences on Lying

The evidence for deceptive behaviors in lower species, as reviewed above, is convincing. The stereotypical nature of many of these behaviors suggests that they are controlled by instincts and, thus, by genetic factors. Is it possible that lying in humans might be influenced by heredity? There is some support for this theory. Bond and Robinson (1988) reviewed prior research studies and concluded that biological factors contribute to human deception, that family members have similarities in types and patterns of lying, and that these similarities result from shared genes. The studies on which these opinions were based had methodological flaws, but they provide some suggestive data nonetheless.

A very large Hawaiian family (3,121 members) was studied through a number of self-report personality inventories (Ahern et al. 1982). Of the more than 50 personality traits evaluated, the strongest (by far) kinship relationship was for lying. This finding must be interpreted with caution because a kinship relationship for behavioral characteristics is not necessarily due to heredity. Environmental, cultural, and child-rearing techniques could also contribute to shared characteristics. Furthermore, the method used to evaluate lying was the lie scale of the Eysenck Personality Inventory (EPI). This scale measures the degree to which a person answers questions in an effort to present a good impression. Although suggestive of deception, an elevated EPI lie score is not directly equivalent to everyday lying.

More direct evidence of hereditary influence comes from a multifactorial study of 265 twin pairs. Rowe (1986) investigated several potential causes of delinquency and found that general environmental factors, such as social class or child-rearing styles, were not influential. Significant factors did include the intrafamily environment (e.g., perceived parental rejection) and genetics. Of the genetic influences, the principal correlates were deceitfulness and temperamental traits.

Bond and Robinson (1988) hypothesized that the genetic factors controlling anatomy also influence lying. They suggest that some people look more honest than others and thus can lie more effectively. As a result of successful deceit, they receive reinforcement and progressively become better liars. However, heredity also influences neurophysiological processes as well as anatomy. It seems probable that genetic influences on cognitive style (see above), neurocognitive impairment, and the propensity to use repression as a coping mechanism (see Chapter 2) might better explain any hereditary predisposition to lying.

Summary

Deceit is a common, basic characteristic of life in the animal kingdom. It is such a potent factor in survival that its expression has evolved independently in many phyla, as flight has evolved in insects, birds, and mammals. It has been suggested that the evolution of the human brain was driven by pressures for ever-increasing cognitive skills at perpetrating and detecting deceit. Furthermore, self-deception may also have evolved as a result of the role it plays in increasing the effectiveness of other-deception. Suggestive evidence points to the possibility of hereditary influences on the propensity to lie.

The human brain is organized into specialized, somewhat independent but interacting, functional entities. The prefrontal lobes appear to be critical for discerning subtle meanings of information regarding social relationships. Thus, defects in the frontal lobes or functional disconnections of various areas of the brain may explain some types of deceit (e.g., unintentionally making statements one knows to be false) or self-deception.

A provocative hypothesis is that the inherent survival advantages of deceit are modulated by social group pressures and an internal system of checks and balances. Thus, higher cortical functions make a person a more effective liar because of the capacity to read the subtle cues of the intended target. With dysfunction of these higher functions, lying becomes cruder, more easily detected, and recognized as pathological. Finally, differences among confabulation, pseudologia fantastica, and possibly the hysterical cognitive style may be quantitative rather than qualitative.

Chapter 4

Learning to Lie: Developmental Issues in Deceit

Lying has its normative functions as well as its pathology and so does telling the truth.

—Arnold Goldberg

Most people are not, despite the common phrase, "born liars"; rather, there is a developmental process by which an individual learns how to lie. The concepts of truth-telling and of lying are inexorably intertwined; each requires the other because one cannot lie without knowledge of the truth. Furthermore, a child can neither lie nor tell the truth without having reached a certain level of maturity in terms of cognitive processes. Some degree of reality testing must be present, and secondary thought processes must be sufficiently developed in order to distinguish between the inner world and the outer world (A. Freud 1965). Lying also requires an awareness of the concept of deception. How does one get another person to believe something different from the "truth"?

Developmental Stages

For the purposes of this review, I arbitrarily divided the developmental stages of lying into three stages, although obviously each overlaps with the others. These stages are 1) early childhood, approximately ages 2–6 years; 2) latency, approximately ages 6–12 years; and 3) adolescence, approximately ages 12–18 years. Furthermore, any discussion of a developmental process must consider the environment in which it occurs. No individual develops (matures) outside of a social milieu, and no individual is unaffected by environmental events. Therefore, I also consider child-rearing styles, the social milieu, and the relevance of extraordinary (traumatic) events.

Early Childhood

The age at which children can truly lie is a continuing topic of debate. To avoid using the word "lie," other language (e.g., false utterance or pseudo-lie) has been used to describe various forms of deceptive behaviors of small children (Sodian 1991). It has been proposed that to genuinely lie, a child must have a concept of the beliefs of other people. A lie represents a deliberate intent to induce a false belief in another person. The concept of another person's mind (as opposed to the state of infantile narcissism) does not develop until at least age 3½ years, according to some investigators (LaFreniere 1988; Sodian 1991). These theorists interpret deceptive-appearing behaviors that occur at earlier ages as efforts by the child to be socially pleasing (compliant) with authoritarian adults or as learned behavior responses to avoid punishment.

Leekam (1992) described three levels of lying, each of which requires an increasingly sophisticated social awareness in association with cognitive maturation. The first level is that of manipulating the behavior of another person. A young child might deny a misdeed or blame another child with the hope of avoiding punishment or social disapproval yet have no intent of influencing another person's belief. On the second level of lying, the child considers the beliefs of another person and intends to manipulate these beliefs.

This ability to conceptualize another person's beliefs enables the child to become more successful at deceit. The child also recognizes that the target of the lie will evaluate any future statement in the light of the new belief. The third level of lying takes into account the listener's evaluation of the liar's intent and sincerity about the lie. It is important that the listener believes the content of what is being said. Thus, there is an awareness of one's nonverbal behavior and a capacity to gauge the level of the listener's credulity. This feedback system allows considerable increase in the ability to provide credible stories.

Woolf (1949) stated that children cannot lie before age 4 years because they do not know the truth. He stated that after age 5 years, the concept of lying becomes clear, and the child has a greater ability to distinguish external reality from fantasy. Woolf's determination of the age at which deceit may first appear has been challenged. LaFreniere (1988) reported anecdotal descriptions of deceitful behavior in children as early as age 19 months. LaFreniere interpreted deceit at this age to be humorous, to provoke laughter, and to maintain attention. An example of this was my experience of playing a game with my then 19-month-old son. He was identifying animals in a picture book and repeatedly gave me the wrong name for a zebra, calling it a giraffe. He then laughed uproariously at my attempts to teach him the correct name. LaFreniere also described situations in which a 2-year-old boy blamed his brother (who was not present) for spilling milk and a 2½-year-old girl who bit herself and then indicated that another child had done it to her.

Dr. Michael Lewis and his colleagues (1989) at the Institute for the Study of Child Development, Robert Wood Johnson Medical School in New Jersey, reported a very interesting experiment in which 3-year-old children (while being videotaped through a one-way mirror) were told not to look at a toy. The experimenter would leave the room and then return in 5 minutes to ask whether the child had looked at the toy. Eighty-five percent of the children disobeyed and peeked at the toy, but only 38% admitted to having done so; some children who had looked refused to answer the question. More girls than boys showed deceptive behavior, and their deceptiveness was more difficult to detect than that of the boys. Interestingly, those children who did lie demonstrated more smiling and relaxed faces than those who told the truth, irrespective of whether they had peeked. Those children who refused to answer (all of whom had actually peeked) showed an increase in anxious touching, thereby demonstrating that their skill in deception was less developed than in those who could be verbally deceptive.

By using experimental "hide-and-seek" games played with small children, researchers have shown that children as young as 2½ years can consciously attempt to deceive others. Chandler and colleagues (1989) of the University of British Columbia reported that their young subjects "not only slyly lied and disingenuously misled, but did so with what often amounted to disarming delight in leading others astray" (p. 1275).

The fantasy lie is characteristic of young and immature children and those older children who regress in response to acute stress or intolerable situations (A. Freud 1965). The child who tells fantasy lies at an early age may talk about wishes as if they were true (e.g., possessions or trips to Disneyland, particularly if a peer has the desired toy or experience).

Several authors have suggested that lying is an essential part of psychic development (Goldberg 1973; Kohut 1966; Tausk 1933). Separation from the parents, particularly the mother, is an important developmental task and occurs not only physically but also in the psychic structure. At what point do one's own ego boundaries end and another's begin? For the young child, the inevitable internal questions are: "Am I my own person?" "Am I a part of my mother?" "Can she read my mind?"

Lying becomes an important, perhaps essential, mechanism by which children can test the limits of their own ego boundaries in order to define themselves and establish autonomy. If a child tells a lie and the mother acts as if the child were truthful, it is evident that the mother cannot control the child's thinking or know the child's thoughts. Thus, lying is one means to differentiate and separate oneself in an effort to establish a distinct and individual identity. Tausk (1933), writing about a child's first lies, said: "The striving for the right to have secrets from which the parents are excluded is one of the most powerful factors in the formation of the ego, especially in establishing and carrying out one's own will" (p. 67). Ekstein and Caruth (1972) expanded this concept, proposing that genuine intimacy rests on the ability to simultaneously maintain and share secrets.

Heinz Kohut (1966) offered further proposals regarding the psychic importance of lying by a child. He suggested that the undetected lie of a child reveals to the child a shortcoming in the idealized omniscient parent. In other words, if children can successfully lie to their parents, then the parents are not really as powerful as previously imagined. Kohut (1966) further proposed that the lost quality of parental omniscience is incorporated as a part of the individual's internalized controls (self-discipline) and becomes " . . . a significant aspect of the all-seeing eye, the omniscience of the super ego" (p. 249).

These ideas suggest in very different ways that if the parent is perceived as not all-powerful and therefore unable to protect and control the child, then the child must develop his or her own mechanism for self-control.

Thus, in addition to being a developmental issue related to separation or autonomy, lying may play a developmental role in the growth of self-regulation.

Latency

Developmental issues in early childhood revolve largely around relationships with parents, self-differentiation and autonomy, and the rudimentary concepts of right and wrong (i.e., the origins of a conscience, or in psychoanalytic terms, a *superego*). When children begin to attend school, they must learn new tasks. These tasks include establishing interpersonal relationships that extend beyond the family and defining one's relationship to society at large. The process of socialization evolves as children are taught, both directly and indirectly, acceptable modes of behavior. The children also begin to experience conflicts between the values and "truth" taught in the family home and those expressed by other elements of society. They learn that the family's "truth" is not necessarily shared by everyone. Furthermore, intimate details of the family, which have been communicated with both overt and subtle messages, must be kept secret. Thus, latency is the time when children learn how to communicate, what not to communicate, and how to deceive.

Much of our knowledge about children's capacity to deceive is derived from the work of experimental psychologists. For example, one research strategy (R. S. Feldman et al. 1979) was to give research subjects of varying ages drinks that tasted either good or bitter. The subjects were told to convince adult observers, who did not know which drink the subject received, that all the drinks tasted good, regardless of the actual taste. The results were clear-cut. The first graders' efforts to deceive failed because their facial expressions gave them away. Seventh graders were more successful, and they typically used a strategy in which they attempted to look just as pleased when the drink tasted bad as when it tasted good. College students enjoyed performing; they appeared to like the bad-tasting drinks even more than the good-tasting drinks.

This experiment demonstrated that an important component of deceit depends not only on the words used but also on control of one's nonverbal communications, including facial expressions and body movements. Six- and 7-year-old children had learned how to lie with words but did not have sufficient control of their nonverbal behaviors to be effective deceivers. With increasing age and experience, a child learns how to monitor these other channels of communication and how to send false nonverbal messages in addition to false words. Other research (R. S. Feldman and White 1980) indicated that children's attempts at successful facial deception may be accompanied by unsuccessful bodily concealment (and vice versa). This is further evidence that children are limited in the use of their various channels for communication and mechanisms for deceit.

B. M. DePaulo and Jordan (1982) proposed that with the progressive development of more finely tuned communicative capabilities, both verbal and nonverbal, effective liars may learn first how to monitor the listener (the target of the lie) carefully for signs of skepticism and then how to modify the message accordingly. Such sophistication requires the capacity to read subtle, often nonverbal, messages from another person (feedback) and then alter one's own communications.

B. M. DePaulo and Jordan (1982) stated that verbally oriented strategies of deceit include denial, distortion, evasiveness, nonresponsiveness, fabrication, irrelevance, and omission of essential facts. They suggested that denial (e.g., "No, I didn't eat the cookies!") may be the simplest of these strategies, and thus, it may appear early in development. These authors also stated that lies come in many varieties and that different types may appear at different developmental points. They suggested that lies aimed at attaining material benefits may appear earlier than does deceit to secure more subtle social rewards. For example, a 4-year-old girl who had been promised freshly baked brownies after her toys were put away soon returned with the claim that she had done so. A quick inspection confirmed the suspicion that little or no progress had been made. Lies told to avoid punishment (or to blame someone else) appear later; most small children (before age 4 or 5 years) will admit what they have done. For example, the 3-year-old brother of a screaming infant will generally answer truthfully when asked, "Did you hit him?" By age 5 or 6 years, the child's answers may not be "truthful." Loyalty lies (lies to protect a friend) occur developmentally somewhat later, and DePaulo and Jordan suggest that they probably predate truly altruistic lies, such as taking blame oneself or accepting punishment rather than implicating a friend.

Braginsky (1970) described some characteristics and techniques of children who lie skillfully. As part of a sophisticated research design, the investigator presented herself to fifth graders as a representative of a cracker company. She gave these 10-year-old children a taste of a cracker that had been dipped in a bitter-tasting quinine solution and then offered the children a nickel for every cracker they could get an unsuspecting peer to eat. Children whose personalities were more manipulative (as measured by scores on a test for Machiavellianism—a manipulative approach to interpersonal relationships) were more successful in getting their peers to eat the bitter-tasting crackers. They engaged in a variety of behaviors that included omissive lies, commissive lies, bribery, two-sided arguments, and transferal of blame to the experimenter. Furthermore, evaluators who listened to tape recordings of the children's conversations with peers rated the manipulative children as sounding more innocent, calmer, and more comfortable than the less manipulative children. These manipulative children were also thought to use more effective (although not necessarily more honest) arguments.

In this experiment, manipulative girls told different kinds of lies from those of manipulative boys. The girls more often told omissive lies (i.e., they withheld information and evaded questions), and the boys more frequently told commissive lies (i.e., they distorted information). For each gender, the strategy was appropriate, insofar as omissive lies worked better for the girls than for the boys, and commissive lies worked better for the boys than for the girls. These results were similar to those described for adult liars, as reported by B. M. DePaulo and colleagues (1982b). The investigators found that women who are lying are more likely than men who are lying to make comments that are less judgmental and more neutral (more evasive and noncommittal) than when they are telling the truth.

When they participate and develop skills in sports and games, latency-age children are actively "taught" how to deceive. In fact, organized sports and games are training grounds for increasing skills in deception. For example, in sports such as basketball and football, players are taught to "fake" movements, including those of the eyes, in order to fool the opposition about which direction a ball will be thrown. Card games such as Old Maid teach children how to control their emotions and facial movements in order to disguise the location of the Old Maid card. Board games such as checkers and chess teach the child how not to signal elation or disappointment in response to an opponent's moves. In fact, skillful players may learn to send false signals (see discussion of poker players in Chapter 10).

Although uncensored truth-telling in a small child may be cute—"Grandma, your hat looks funny!"—the latency-age child is often encouraged not to tell the truth in such situations. Furthermore, the concepts of social customs and "white lies" are introduced (often simultaneously with proscriptions against lying). The child is told not to say anything that will embarrass someone else (including the nuclear family), even if it is true. Family matters such as sex, money, and substance abuse are particular areas of discretion and deception. Woe unto the boy who publicly comments about his mother's or his father's hair-coloring activities! Family secrets such as alcoholism must be maintained. In families with "dark secrets" (e.g., sexual, physical, or substance abuse), much of the family energy is spent in deceptive behaviors in order to maintain a facade of social propriety (Saarni and von Salisch 1993). As a consequence, latency-age children may be introduced to mental "double book-keeping" activities in order to keep part of their knowledge out of public view, even if it requires considerable deceit. To some degree, double bookkeeping occurs in all families, but for most it may only involve secrecy about mother's or father's hair dye or the parents' argument about how much money was spent on the last vacation.

During latency, children learn to lie effectively and to take their place in society. According to Marie Vasek (1986), a psychologist who has studied the development of lying in children, "The skills required in deception are also used in being compassionate and co-ordinating our actions with those of others, and without them human society might not exist" (p. 291).

Adolescence

During adolescence, the early childhood conflicts about lying and truth-telling are reactivated. The psychic stresses encountered during adolescence (e.g., separation issues, sexual drives, and behavior) may result in a fragmentation of the self, which leads to lying as a symptom (Goldberg 1973). Adolescents and their parents may be in a quandary about what to communicate to each other. Adolescents may view their parents as hypocritical, corrupt, or deceitful. Simultaneously, the adolescents' struggles about their own separation from the control and protection of parents often reactivate behaviors such as secrecy and deceit in the effort to become an autonomous person. Adolescents may also overreact to their own fears of lying or their parents' dissimulations, indulging in "pathological truth-telling." This may be manifested as excessive scrupulosity as adolescents attempt to become more familiar with their internal regulatory mechanisms. Goldberg (1973) said, in describing adolescence, that "no period better demonstrates the idea that lying is as much a part of normal growth and development as is telling the truth" (p. 108). He goes on to "suspect that one of the turning points from adolescence to adulthood is learning that openness often is cruelty and saying whatever is in one's mind is an indulgence that no adult can afford" (p. 111).

Learning the Morality of Deceit

Another developmental task related to deception and truthfulness is determining the morality of lying. Is it right or wrong to tell a lie? The pioneer investigator in this area was the Swiss psychologist Jean Piaget. Piaget (1932/1965) viewed the child's propensity to tell lies as a natural tendency, "so spontaneous and universal that we can take it as an essential part of the child's egocentric thought" (p. 139). In the child, therefore, the problem of lies is the clash of the egocentric attitude with the moral constraint of the adult. Piaget's investigations revealed that young children, about age 6 years, equate swearing (naughty words) with lying; to tell a lie is to commit a moral fault by means of language. Children in this age range, although able to make a distinction between an intentional misrepresentation and an involuntary mistake, do not emphasize the distinction and consider both as lies. The identification of mistakes as lies disappears at about age 8 years, but it is not until about age 10 years that lying is explicitly defined as an intentionally false statement.

Young children (e.g., age 6 years) also judge the moral magnitude of a lie by its deviation from credibility rather than by the malignancy of its content. For example, children at this age would regard a girl who said that she saw a dog as big as a cow as "naughtier" than a girl who lied about her school grades. Similarly, a lie is regarded by young children as more serious if it accompanies actions that have material ill effects (e.g., spilling a can of paint). Also, lies are often judged by younger children primarily by their concrete consequences; they are bad because one is punished for them.

Piaget believed that by age 10 or 11 years, children have developed the ability to regard the intent of the lie to deceive as the primary moral issue rather than its overt content. He interpreted this change as the result of the child's ability to move away from the egocentric position, in which a tendency is to alter the truth and neglect reality in accordance with desires.

True autonomy requires seeing other people as separate and regarding truthfulness (now internalized as a value) as necessary for mutual respect and intimacy.

The work of Piaget has stimulated other investigators to study the moral meaning of lying in children. Wimmer and colleagues (1985) found that the moral intuition of young children (age 4–5 years) is quite advanced compared with their definitions of lying. In other words, their sense of right and wrong in regard to the truth is developed to a greater extent than their linguistic capacity to define a lie. Peterson and colleagues (1983) showed videotaped stories depicting deliberate lies and unintentional untrue statements to subjects who varied in age from 5 years to adulthood. These investigators' update of Piaget's 1932 work confirmed many of his general findings, even though some differences were found. They concluded that the harsh moral evaluations of lies exhibited by young children tended to become more lenient with a transition to adulthood. Also, to some extent, all age groups judged selfishly motivated lies to be worse than unintended misstatements. The investigators also found that although younger children cited the prohibition against lying as originating from the punitive sanctions of authority, older children were more likely to see the prohibition in terms of fairness and its effect on trust.

One major difference between the findings of Peterson and colleagues and those of Piaget was that the former group found that the transition of attitudes toward lying was much more gradual among age groups and that younger children (e.g., age 5 years) often had a greater capacity to evaluate the self-serving functions and moral implications of lies than Piaget had concluded. These differences may have reflected differences in 1) culture over a 50-year period, 2) methodological factors, or 3) interpretation of the data (e.g., Wimmer and colleagues [1985] disagreed with Piaget about the interpretation of the latter's data).

A study (Bussey 1992) of Australian children's evaluations of truth and lying found that about 70% of preschool children could accurately distinguish between truthful statements and lies. This percentage increased with age, and by age 11 years virtually all children were accurate in their judgments of truthfulness. Of note, however, Bussey found that young children (ages 4 and 5 years) were more likely to attempt to avoid lying than to actively seek to tell the truth, especially if they expected punishment for truthfulness. That is, a young child's motivation not to lie is fear rather than an internalized positive value for truthfulness. Older children (ages 8–11 years) were able to ascribe pride to truthfulness. Bussey proposed that successful socialization results in a transfer from external forms of control to internal controls and that this occurs in the developmental period of early latency.

Impression Management

Erving Goffman (1959) in his book, *The Presentation of Self in Everyday Life*, now regarded as a classic work in social psychology, used the metaphor of the theater to describe peoples' efforts to present themselves to others. In a sense, the whole world is a stage on which we manage our self-representations to others in order to convey the impressions that we wish them to have about us. Many of these representations are determined by societal expectations (rules). Some are prescribed roles that we play, and others are efforts to deceive. Thus, a sales agent will continue to be polite and gracious even after spending a lengthy time with a potential customer who does not make a purchase; a physician appears to be confident and self-assured, even when perplexed about a patient's medical problem; and a customer who actually wishes to purchase an automobile may feign disinterest in it, with the hope of being in a better position to negotiate a favorable price. Although there may be considerable variation or skill, by adulthood essentially everyone has developed skills that permit discrepancies between experienced internal thoughts and feelings and those displayed to the external world.

Dr. Carolyn Saarni of Sonoma State University, California, has been a leading investigator of how and when children learn to regulate and dissimulate their emotional expressions (Saarni 1979, 1982; Saarni and von Salisch 1993). She found that by age 6 years, children have some concept of what is appropriate in terms of emotional expressiveness and that this understanding increases with age. Children learn that a direct and open expression of their emotions may make them more vulnerable, result in loss of self-esteem, violate cultural norms, or hurt the feelings of others.

Saarni (1984) studied emotional dissimulation by using the research technique of giving an age-inappropriate toy to children of varied ages and carefully recording their emotional responses. The socially appropriate response to a gift is pleasure, regardless of one's true feelings. Six-year-old children, particularly boys, openly expressed their dismay at receiving a baby toy. By age 10 or 11 years, most children, especially girls, responded positively to the gifts, even though secretly they certainly must have been disappointed.

Effective deceit is largely determined by the consistency and sincerity of nonverbal communication. It is reasonable to assume that the social skills associated with emotional dissimulation (playing the appropriate social role at the proper time) will translate into increased skill in lying (Saarni 1982).

Child-Rearing Styles

Although differences in neurophysiology (see Chapter 3) among individuals may account for differences in their propensity to tell the truth, there can be little doubt that parental and cultural factors influence the degree to which children lie (Smith 1968). For example, how did the parents respond to the young child's initial lies? Was there severe punishment? Were the lies ignored? Were they regarded as cute? Similarly, were the child's fantasies indiscriminately encouraged or severely suppressed, or did the parents help the child to recognize the difference between creative fantasy and reality?

A variety of studies have indicated that a major reason for childhood lying is to avoid negative consequences. Therefore, Stouthamer-Loeber (1986) suggested that children who have very punitive parents may have more to gain by lying and, as a result, may establish a pattern of lying. Children who score high in features of Machiavellianism have been reported to regard other individuals as persons to be deceived, disobeyed, and manipulated. Furthermore, the emergence of Machiavellianism has been correlated with rejection of, or disappointment in, the parents as appropriate role models (Touhey 1973). In contrast, parents who regard lying and truthfulness as something to teach their children may spend more constructive time with them, thereby influencing behavior in a more positive direction.

It is reasonable to assume that the different ways parents respond to their children's prevarications and fantasies extinguish or reinforce certain types of verbal behavior and that the patterns, once established, may persist throughout life. Sissela Bok (1978b) warned against excessive paternalistic protection of children from painful truths. She suggested that what a child learns from paternalistic lies is that adults bend the truth when it suits them. On the other hand, she said that those dour parents who fear the unreality of fiction and fairy tales in their children's lives stifle every expression of imagination, at crushing costs to their children and themselves.

The Truthful-Deceitful Social Milieu

Equally important as the response of parents and others to the child's lies and fantasies is the degree to which the child is exposed to lying by others. Are promises made to the child repeatedly broken? Do the parents continuously lie to the child? For example, do they say that they are taking the child to the movies when they are really going to the dentist? Are there many secrets in the household? Are certain aspects of the parents' past lives suppressed or distorted? Is there hypocrisy in the practice of religious customs or in the observance of laws? Are subjects such as Santa Claus presented as myth or as fact? The list is almost endless, and to some extent no family is ever entirely truthful, but we can readily observe the variances among different families.

One woman (see Chapter 6), whose adult life was characterized by habitual lying, learned when she was an adolescent that her father (a fundamentalist Protestant who had frequently railed against sexual promiscuity and divorce) was having an affair and that her mother had been previously married. Furthermore, the myth of Santa Claus (an interesting paradox in view of her father's professed religious views) had been elaborately played out during her childhood. The parents' charade was complete: they left milk and cookies for Santa Claus in the evening, and an empty glass and crumbs were seen on Christmas morning. She was 6 years old when she learned from a classmate that Santa Claus did not exist. This woman regarded the discovery of her mother's prior divorce and her disillusionment about Santa Claus as two of the most traumatic events of her life.

Healy and Healy (1915) reported the cases of two individuals for whom pathological lying seemed at least in part due to the contagion from long continued lying in their home environment. In one case, the patient's marked improvement was attributed to escape from the lying milieu. In a different clinical situation, involving the treatment of a teenage girl for habitual lying, the girl's father had been identified by the mother as a compulsive liar. In one important and amusing episode, the girl had missed a psychotherapy appointment. The mother called the psychotherapist later and asked whether the appointment had been kept. When told it had been missed, the mother said, "I thought so. I was going through her purse and found the appointment card. What do I do now? What story can I make up to let her know that I know about the missed appointment?" When advised by the therapist to be truthful and tell her how she had discovered the appointment card, the mother's response was: "I could never do that!"

The culture and subculture to which a person belongs may also reflect attitudes toward behaviors such as lying. A subculture has been defined as a pattern of values, norms, and behaviors that have become traditional among occupations, ethnic groups, social classes, persons in closed institutions, and different age cohorts. Adolescents, because of peer pressure and their wish to be accepted by peer groups, are particularly sensitive to the values of their groups (subcultures).

In one adolescent gang subculture, six concerns or ideas were identified: trouble, toughness, smartness, excitement, fate, and autonomy (W. B. Miller et al. 1961). Smartness was specifically defined as the ability to dupe or con others successfully. Such an outlook extols the virtues of clever deceit and regards it as shameful to be so incompetent as to be caught in a lie. As a result, these adolescents receive positive reinforcement for deceitful behaviors that occur outside the group. Although skill in lying can be valued in intergroup relationships, duplicity is not conducive to group survival, and intragroup deception is usually proscribed. The Junior Outlaws, a Chicago street gang, shares with the Boy Scout oath the common value of trustworthiness to one another (W. B. Miller et al. 1961). Thus, a person can be caught between the conflicting values of the larger society and those of his or her subculture. In another example, a prisoner might face a conflict in lying to those who are fellow prisoners versus lying to nonconvicts (McGivern 1982).

Role of Traumatic Experiences

The environment in which a child is raised may be so emotionally, physically, or intellectually overwhelming that he or she must use primitive defenses to deal with it. For example, one hypothesis about the origin of multiple personality disorder revolves around the idea that dissociation is one solution to an overwhelmingly traumatic childhood (Coons and Milstein 1986). Similarly, it can be hypothesized that lying can become a way of concealing and ultimately denying that which cannot be assimilated in other ways; lying then serves to support repression or denial. This tentative formulation is consistent with the observations of Fenichel (1954) and with the phenomenological evidence that patients with pseudologia fantastica often report chaotic, inconsistent, and traumatic childhoods (see Chapters 7 and 8). In her description of impostors, Greenacre (1958a) noted that many adult impostors had one specific form of childhood trauma—the father's death during their early childhood.

Pathological Lying in Childhood

Lying has been repeatedly rated as one of the most distressing behaviors of children that concerns parents (Ziv 1970). The lay press, especially magazines targeted toward parenting, frequently publishes articles on the subject or advice from authorities on how to deal with lying. In one study that involved lower-socioeconomic-class subjects, lying was regarded by parents to be of more urgency for intervention than were aggressive behaviors (Alston 1980).

From the discussion above, it is apparent that all children lie and that lying is to a large extent sanctioned, taught, and encouraged by those with whom the child comes in contact. Yet, despite this ambiguity of the definition of deceitful behaviors, some children are labeled as liars. Because all children are, to some degree, liars, why are some children singled out and identified as such? Is it the quantity or quality of the lies, or is it some other distinguishing feature of the child? In her review of many studies, Stouthamer-Loeber (1986) consistently found that children who were referred to mental health centers for conduct disorders were much more likely than average to be labeled as liars by teachers and parents. In contrast, children referred for neurotic disorders were less likely than average to be identified as liars.

In one research study of lying, teachers assessed their fourth-, seventh-, and tenth-grade male students for their propensity to lie (Stouthamer-Loeber and Loeber 1986). Lying was generally rated as occurring less frequently among the older boys. (However, in view of the discussion above about the socialization aspects of lying, it may be that the boys were becoming more skillful at disguising their deceit.) About 3.5% of the boys, at all three age levels, were rated by the teachers as rarely or almost never honest. Among boys of all ages, lying was significantly related to several other problem behaviors such as delinquency, theft, and fighting. These correlations were higher for older children than for younger children. Of importance, children who lied were more likely to come either from homes where mothers or fathers poorly supervised or rejected their children or from homes where parents did not get along well or did not live together. Socioeconomic status was not related to lying.

The investigators of the above study questioned whether lying was a by-product of other problem behaviors or whether it was the basis for the development of increasingly more delinquent behaviors. In other words, is lying a developmental step in the process that produces thieves? Yet another possibility is that lying and delinquency may have common origins. Along this line of reasoning, the poor parental contact described above might lead to poor socialization, which results in antisocial behaviors and lies in an attempt to avoid punishment. Children who have more parental involvement might learn to lie in more socially accepted modes.

The label of *chronic liar* is a warning sign for problems emerging later in life. Stouthamer-Loeber (1986) concluded that chronic childhood lying is significantly correlated with the development of maladjustment in later life, including drug and alcohol use and aggressive offenses. It must be recognized that despite these statistical correlations, many children who lie do not have such morbid outcomes. However, Stouthamer-Loeber found no studies in her review that suggested that chronic lying in childhood led to the later development of close personal ties.

Summary

Lying in children is a normal phenomenon that occurs in association with learning how to tell the truth. Lying is, in the view of many authorities, an essential component in the process of developing autonomy and differentiating oneself from one's parents. The capacity to fool parents demonstrates to children that the parents are not omniscient and omnipotent; therefore, children must discard the fantasy that they will always have an all-powerful protector. In relinquishing these fantasies, children must accept certain responsibilities for the care and protection of themselves, thus facilitating the development of both ego and superego functions.

The process of learning how to lie is influenced by child-rearing practices and the social milieu in which the child is raised; that is, lying is reinforced (positively or negatively) by the degree to which the child is rewarded or punished for deceitful behavior. There appear to be distinctive differences in family and other subculture units in the degree to which lying occurs on a daily basis. If the child experiences repeated trauma (e.g., sexual abuse, physical abuse, or being raised in a family with an alcoholic parent), lying may become one way to cope with stress. Certainly, putting on a false face appears to be one coping mechanism learned when growing up in a family involved with alcoholism.

Finally, it appears that learning to lie in social situations—the white lie of social interchange—is associated with greater skill in interpersonal relationships and may be regarded as a sign of sophistication. Learning how and when to lie and how and when to tell the truth are major developmental tasks.

Chapter 5

Why People Lie: The Determinants of Deceit

The most common lie is the lie one tells to oneself.

—Nietzsche

In the preceding chapters, I have examined many factors that influence behavior and may predispose a person to telling a lie. From this material, it is obvious that everyone lies; the difference among people is in the frequency, target, and degree of those lies. In this chapter, I address various factors that influence the process of lying itself. Why do some people lie when the truth would serve them better? In these situations, it seems that the content of the lie is not as important as the telling of the lie itself. I review some general aspects of motivation and explore in greater detail some specific factors that determine motivation for deceit. These factors can lead to the occasional or situational lie of a "normal" person, or they can be so pervasively present as to cause compulsive deceptive behavior that affects the entire personality.

Factors That Influence Motivation for Lying

The various themes discussed in this chapter have, to a large extent, been anticipated by the previous chapter dealing with development. If, in the process of normal development, one fails to master a developmental task, psychological "fixation" at that level is possible. Behaviors that are appropriate for a particular developmental stage (age) may persist into adult life. Furthermore, no person ever completely masters all developmental tasks and, therefore, "normal" persons may regress and use more primitive defenses at times of stress or conflict. Ego mechanisms reflect responses to—as well as attempts to influence—a situation, environment, or event. Motivation is often a complex blend of conscious responses to reality issues and unconscious factors that may reflect underlying conflicts. Any behavior frequently has more than one determinant, and thus more than one of the issues discussed below may be operating at the same time.

Lies to Avoid Punishment

Among the lies that emerge early in childhood are those that are attempts to avoid punishment (e.g., "No, I didn't eat any cookies." "I didn't hit my brother."). This reason for lying continues into adulthood (e.g., "Officer, I was only driving 2 or 3 miles per hour over the speed limit." "I was in the backyard practicing my golf swing at the time my wife was knifed to death.").

Lies to Preserve a Sense of Autonomy

One of the important developmental tasks—separation and individuation—may be associated with lying; through their ability to deceive their parents, children learn that their parents cannot control their (the children's) thinking. Later in life, people who react strongly to control or intrusiveness from others may resort to lying in an effort to maintain a sense of independence. One illustration of this was C. G. Jung's lies to Sigmund Freud in response to the latter's persistent questions about a dream that Jung had described.

Jung deliberately provided inaccurate associations to the dream so that Freud could not accurately analyze it and make an interpretation. This deceit served, in part, to prevent regression in Jung and allowed his further self-delineation as an independent thinker (Winnicott 1964).

A less esoteric example is that of a young lawyer who repeatedly engaged in extramarital affairs. His behavior had a compulsive quality about it, yet, on close examination in psychotherapy, it appeared that the behavior was less determined by sexuality than by other psychological purposes. This young man did not have an exceptionally high sexual drive nor did he obtain much sexual gratification from his affairs. Furthermore, his wife was both attractive and sexually available. In many respects, he described his sexual relationship with her as more satisfying than those with the women whom he was seeing clandestinely. However, one important aspect of his relationship with his wife was that she reminded him of his mother, who was very controlling and intrusive. In fact, his wife had also attempted to control many aspects of his life, including issues such as which church he should attend. Through the process of psychotherapy, it became apparent that this young man was using his sexual liaisons as a means of maintaining a secret life and a sense of autonomous maleness. A response to his wife's controlling and intrusive behavior, his affairs served to counteract his feeling of being a "little boy." His deceitful behavior, including overt lies to cover his tracks, was motivated less by erotic excitement than by the need for psychological independence.

Lies as an Act of Aggression

In our society, one of the most infuriating feelings comes from the realization that one has been lied to. There is often a sense of being devalued, insulted, and betrayed. It follows, then, that lying, if it is perceived by the recipient as an injury, may be perpetrated as an aggressive act. One may lie to another person with a belief that the other does not deserve the truth and with a feeling of contempt that the other is not smart enough to decipher the lie. Bursten (1972) described this as achieving a feeling of superiority by "putting something over" on another person. Thus, lies can be conceived as a form of verbal aggression or sadism.

An example of this type of behavior is that of a corporate vice president who repeatedly lied. He actively and vigorously recruited senior managers from other companies around the country to his own division and promised them increased responsibilities, salary, clerical support, and other enticements. On arrival at their new jobs, each of these new recruits discovered that the promises could not or would not be fulfilled. Apologies were accompanied by a series of slickly offered rationalizations. Rage on the part of the new manager would inevitably follow, and an awkward period of readjustment for the entire division would occur. The broken promises were, on the whole, unnecessary, and they inevitably led to more problems than a truthful, straightforward approach would have brought. Examination of the deceitful vice president's own childhood background revealed that his father was irresponsible and frequently left the family for extended periods of time. It seems reasonable to hypothesize that the vice president's selective choice of senior managers as targets of deceitful behavior was motivated by unconscious anger toward his father and simultaneous identification with him.

Lies to Obtain a Sense of Power

A basic characteristic of human society is that human relationships and civilization depend on shared accurate information. A person who possesses more information (knowledge) is usually more powerful in controlling both the environment and other persons. The purpose of an education is, in essence, to obtain greater power over the environment and (in a different way) over others in a societal setting. For example, training to be an attorney certainly provides the latter type of power.

If information is associated with power, then one way to affect one's power relationship with other people is to reduce their power by providing them with misinformation or by keeping aspects of one's own information a secret (as may occur in guilds, religious sects, etc.). This phenomenon is clearly seen in international politics; governments attempt to maintain a high level of secrecy about weapons, economics, and industrial research. Furthermore, misinformation is commonly distributed, particularly about military operations and diplomatic moves. If individuals or groups misunderstand their competitors, their power has been reduced. Lying (the transmission of false information) can therefore be seen as a means of increasing one's own power by deliberately decreasing that of another. Misinformation limits the rational choices available to the person to whom a lie has been told.

A word of caution is in order regarding power and lying. Bok (1978a) noted that power derived from lying is effective only insofar as one is believed. Once the liar is recognized as such, his or her information is regarded as suspect; the person who becomes known as a liar may actually lose power (see the related discussion of reciprocal altruism and deceit in Chapter 3).

The previous discussion has been based on a concrete concept of information and power. However, such concrete principles can be extrapolated into unconscious needs. People who feel that they lack power may resort to lying as a way of increasing their sense of power. Initially, they may obtain greater control of their environmental situation and therefore be positively reinforced. With such reinforcement, the behavior is maintained and can be seen as similar to an addiction because of the short-term rewards. In other words, each time a person tells a successful lie, he or she achieves a sense of superiority and power. Such behavior may then be repeated to obtain the same feeling, even when the lie meets no external needs.

A clinical example that illustrates this phenomenon is that of a 5-year-old boy reported by Woolf (1949). The boy's father was away in the army, and his absence left the child with a sense of weakness and vulnerability. Although economic circumstances were favorable, the boy feigned poverty in order to beg for money. From his successful imposture of an impoverished waif, he was able to obtain a feeling of triumphant superiority and power.

Another illustration of this type of underlying motivation is that of a person with a factitious disorder. Persons who simulate a disease and by doing so fool others, including doctors, obtain a sense of control and mastery while simultaneously having their needs for nurturing met (M. D. Feldman and Ford 1994). The phenomenon of medical impostors is detailed in Chapter 8.

Lies for the Delight of Putting One Over

The delight that one may achieve through fooling someone else is one aspect of achieving a sense of power through deceit. The friends of a bright and compulsive, but anxious and insecure, medical intern decided to play a practical joke on him. During one of the intern's first nights of on-call duty, one of the friends disguised his voice and telephoned the intern. This friend pretended to be an out-of-town physician who was transferring an acutely sick patient to the university hospital. He said the patient was in cardiac failure with a rare arrhythmia. He went on to provide a medical history that included renal disease, hepatic failure, and poor diabetic control. With the description of each new medical complication of this medical emergency, the intern's anxiety grew, and his face became paler and paler. Finally, the conspirators, who were secretly watching, could bear it no longer and burst out with laughter. The intern, now realizing he was the butt of a joke, embarrassingly joined the laughter in a good-hearted (if "false-hearted") manner.

Practical jokes, although hilarious to the perpetrators, may not be amusing to the victims. Unlike genuine humor, the practical joke often contains underlying aggression and hostility in the guise of a joke. A thrill is often associated with fooling someone else—a sense of power, cleverness, and superiority. Ekman (1992) coined the phrase *duping delight* to describe this particular form of pleasure in successfully perpetrating a deceit. Bursten (1972) described similar feelings by his use of the term *putting one over*. Duping delight may result from the success of a relatively innocuous practical joke, or it may be a motivational component of more malignant forms of deceit such as con games, imposture, or Munchausen syndrome (see Chapter 8).

Lies as Wish Fulfillment

The wish-fulfillment lie is a common phenomenon in children ages 4–7 years. At this stage in their lives, when reality testing is less well developed, children often confuse a wish with reality. Thus, children often make statements that do not include the preface of "I wish I could," or "I wish that." Children also may be confused by the unconscious belief that if a fantasy is spoken out loud, it might come true. Such statements are usually innocuous and are normal behavior. If parents handle these situations well, they can help their children define the difference between reality and healthy fantasy. As an example of a childlike wish-fulfillment lie, a 5-year-old who wants his father to admire and love him might say, "Daddy, when I grow up I'm going to buy you a great big airplane." "We are going to go to Disney World this summer" is a typical wish-fulfillment lie told by a child whose family's economic circumstances would not allow such a vacation. A 7-year-old boy who wants admiration and acceptance as an athlete from his peers (even though his athletic skills are meager) might falsely tell his friends that his uncle is a major league baseball player.

Wish-fulfillment lies of children are usually normal, but they may persist into adulthood in a much more pathological form. A nurse had purposely created a potentially fatal condition in herself by surreptitiously taking anticancer medications (see Chapter 8). This woman, who had had a deprived and dramatic childhood, also told stories about being the pampered daughter of a wealthy man. She described how, as a teenager, she traveled from horse show to horse show pulling her horses behind her luxurious convertible automobile.

At the borderline between pathological and "normal" lying are the exaggerations frequently used in day-to-day conversations. Such exaggerations may be inflated sales figures reported by a sales agent at a cocktail party or remembrances and descriptions of athletic prowess during college. As described by Helene Deutsch (1921/1982), such stories often develop the quality of a personal myth (see Chapter 13) and, when frequently retold, begin to have the semblance of real memories (see Chapter 9). Davidoff (1942) noted how the fantasy lie provides some sense of gratification, even if only for a short time. Wish-fulfillment lying is often used by persons who lack the ability to sustain the effort required to create or produce accomplishments of their own.

Lies to Assist Self-Deception

Fenichel (1954) suggested that lying is a means of facilitating repression. Fenichel's formulations are supported by Marcos's (1972) report of a patient who lied continuously during psychotherapy. This patient's denial of her pervasive sexual problems served the defensive purpose of preventing the emergence of conflictive material related to her identification with her mother. The mother was also sexually dysfunctional, and the lies prevented the patient from focusing on the painful and undesired recognition of her similarities to the mother.

By definition, lying must be a conscious process; there must be the intent to deceive. Even so, the ratio of conscious and unconscious influences on deceit of oneself and others varies. People use rationalization to explain their behavior or responsibility for certain outcomes, thus disguising from themselves and others the true nature of their underlying drives, needs, and abilities. For example, a young man offered the excuse of antisemitism as the reason he was not accepted to a graduate program in business administration. In truth, both his aptitude scores and his college record were significantly below those of the average student in the program. However, acknowledging that his failures were due to personal inadequacies would have been more painful than seeing himself as the object of prejudicial actions. A young woman conflicted about her sexuality might explain her sexual behavior the previous night by saying she was caught up in romantic love or had had too much champagne. Such explanations help disguise her consciously unacceptable wish for sexual gratification.

As mentioned before, many of the ego-defense mechanisms serve the role of self-deception (see Chapter 2). They may also be used as excuses to other people in an effort to disavow one's own weaknesses and failings.

Lying may displace or disguise conscious awareness of conflict, but ironically it can simultaneously highlight the conflict through the symbolism of the content of the lie. Blum (1983) reported the case of a young man who postponed the beginning of his psychoanalysis with the excuse that his mother had just died, which was not true. She had not died, but the content of the lie proved to be the focal point of the therapy: the patient's ambivalence toward his mother and his unresolved grief over the death of his father during his childhood. Thus, through telling lies, we may attempt to disguise from ourselves certain painful feelings and affects, but through the content of our lies, we simultaneously broadcast to others the very nature of these conflicts.

Lies to Manipulate the Behavior of Others

Lying to have an effect on others is, perhaps, the easiest motivation to understand. No one questions why a person might deny culpability in an effort to avoid punishment; even the lies of a car dealer who is closing a sale are also understandable, if inexcusable. People lie and distort the truth to pursue their own needs and wishes and, at times, the needs of others.

Lies to Help Another Person

The ethical appropriateness of altruistic or paternalistic lies remains an issue of philosophical debate (Bok 1978a). Despite such controversy, concern about other people continues to be a common justification to others (and rationalization to oneself) for telling lies.

The Dutch and Danish people lied about the knowledge of Jews they were hiding. People generally applaud the artistic work of their friends, despite private reservations about its quality. Physicians frequently lie to patients and their families. For example, an emergency room physician might tell the family that the death of their loved one in a car crash was merciful, saying that the victim died instantly without pain, even though the physician knows that death followed a period of agonizing pain.

Most people do not wish to inflict hurt or embarrassment on other people. Deceit, or careful management of the truth, is one of the means used to respect the feelings of others (Nyberg 1993). Bok (1978b) cautioned, however, that the feelings being protected may be one's own. If so, the ostensibly altruistic lie may actually be a self-deceptive lie.

Lies to Accommodate Others' Self-Deception

The liar may, consciously or unconsciously, be lying to help another person maintain self-deception. The basic components of lying are intact: the liar intends to deceive, and the information is known to be false. However, the process of the lie is facilitated by the recipient's willingness, perhaps even eagerness, to be deceived. Some examples will help to clarify this idea.

A woman became suspicious of her husband's sexual fidelity. He had seemingly lost interest in her and frequently left town for business, taking more trips than previously in their marriage. In addition, she smelled a faint but consistent scent of perfume on his clothing. She found a motel receipt that listed two guests for an out-of-town business trip. Although the woman did not want to disrupt the marriage "because of the children" and financial security, when she finally fearfully confronted her husband, he immediately denied any misbehavior and offered glib explanations for her concerns (e.g., "My secretary recently changed her perfume." "Of course, I still love you. I'm just under so much pressure at work."). The wife accepted these answers without question and with an immediate reduction of anxiety. She had been told what she wanted to hear and did not pursue the matter further.

A medical chief of service was told that one of his physicians was inexplicably missing during parts of the workday. Furthermore, that physician had been reported to be occasionally tremulous in the morning, and the smell of alcohol had been detected on his breath. The administrator, who was short-staffed and overworked, reluctantly called the physician to his office and confronted him with the information he had been told. He listened with considerable relief to the explanation that the physician in question might have been using "too much aftershave" and then sent him back to work.

The American people, tired of high taxes and a progressive decline in their standard of living, overwhelmingly elected a presidential candidate who told them that lower taxes would be the engine that would drive a healthier economy and provide a balanced budget.

After carefully studying the game of blackjack, a young physician concluded that a mathematical solution would ensure profitable gambling. While in a casino, he confided to a stranger that he had developed a new system that he believed was foolproof. The stranger told him that the system was "mathematically brilliant" and indicated a willingness to try it using his own money. He steered the young physician to a table and after an hour, profit had accumulated. With this success, the stranger suggested that they make a "real killing." He would arrange financial backing for extensive gambling at another casino, but first he would need some "good faith" money for the backers. The physician gave $1,000 to the man, who was to return in 1 hour; the stranger was never seen again. This common con game relied on the physician's wanting to believe what he was told, namely that he (the "mark") was brilliant and that financial security was imminent. In a different context, this lie would have been disbelieved, but it was now accepted.

A young man, who had enlisted in the navy during the Vietnam era and attended hospital school corps to become a medical corpsman, was referred for psychiatric consultation because of stress and erratic behavior. He explained to the psychiatrist that his behavior was caused by stress and grief related to being drafted into the navy just as he was scheduled to enter medical school. He described in detail his wish to become a physician and his elation at being accepted at a first-rate medical school, only to have these hopes dashed by having to enter military service. The psychiatrist, touched by this story, wrote a sympathetic note on the consultation sheet. Later, a chief petty officer called the psychiatrist and diplomatically questioned the psychiatrist's diagnosis and recommendations. The chief petty officer provided additional information that the man in question was telling stories about combat duty in Vietnam (he had never been out of the continental United States) and other tall tales. He said: "You might want to reevaluate him, Doc." On reexamining the patient, it became apparent that the patient's entire history had been a fabrication. The enlisted man, through pseudologia fantastica, had constructed a story to which the psychiatrist was sympathetic because of the latter's views of the Vietnam War and his own unwelcome military duty. A new consultation report, with different recommendations, was provided for the medical record.

A young naval officer was hospitalized for treatment of his peptic ulcer disease; because his symptoms were unresponsive to the usual medical treatments, psychiatric consultation was requested. The officer reported that he was being "eaten up inside." He was a field intelligence officer whose duty was to obtain information from the hill people of Vietnam. Poor military decisions based on misinformation were resulting in unnecessary loss of life. He stated that his reports would be regularly rewritten to contain inaccurate information and that he would be forced to sign them. He indicated that this procedure occurred up the entire chain of command, and the word was that "heads would roll" if "the man" was not told what he wanted to hear.

In the above example, the careers of naval intelligence officers depended on their willingness to provide false intelligence. They were encouraged to lie to support the self-deception of superiors. These clinical illustrations, reflecting markedly different situations, demonstrate that lying (deception) is often a dynamic process. Both the person who perpetrates the lie (the liar) and the person who accepts it are in collusion to distort the truth. The dependent spouse hears what she wants to believe. The family and supervisors of an alcoholic physician collude with the physician to deny the real problem (a very frequent occurrence in cases of substance abuse). Politicians tell their voting constituencies what the voters want to believe. The con man tells the physician what he wishes to hear. The sympathetic psychiatrist, angry at the war himself, wants to hear of further injustices. Neither one party nor the other has primary blame; rather, deception is a two-way street, a dyadic and dynamic process.

Lies as a Solution to Role Conflict

Individuals who are employees of corporations or members of organizations or religious groups may find conflicting expectations and demands being made on them. Grover (1993a) delineated some of these potential conflicts and suggested that lying and other forms of deceit may be a means of attempting to resolve such role conflicts. One situation described by Grover occurs when the demands of the organization (or employer) are contrary to the individual's personal value system. For example, an employee might be pressured to use sales techniques that he or she believes are offensive or unethical. One solution is for the salesperson to conduct himself or herself in a manner he or she believes proper but to lie to his or her superiors about the behavior, such as how he or she "pressured" a customer to make a sale.

The organizational pressure that occurs when greater or more complex work demands are placed on an employee is also likely to be associated with increased lying. A secretary might say something has been done when it was actually beyond her skill level; a project manager may falsely report that work has been completed. Workers who report to more than one superior are likely to deceive as a means of resolving the conflict of serving two masters. Grover and Hui (1994) found that self-interest (something of tangible benefit to a person) interacted with role conflict in a way that increases the probability of an individual's engaging in deceptive behavior.

Professionals may find their professional values in conflict with the expectations of their employers. For example, a physician employed by a health maintenance organization (whose profits are determined by the amount of medical care *not* provided) might lie about the severity of a patient's symptoms to obtain approval for what the physician believes to be adequate medical care. Not surprisingly, Grover (1993b) found that persons highly committed to their profession were more likely to be accurate in their reports to other members of the same profession than with persons outside their profession. Persons who are highly committed to their organizations are more accurate in their reports to the organization than to persons outside the organization. Grover further observed that lying may be considered ethical behavior in those circumstances in which the organization stands in the way of professional ethical behavior.

The observations of individual behavior in organizations as described above can be generalized to a person's relationship to society at large. We all play many roles, and at times those roles may be contradictory or in conflict. Thus, deceit—either of ourselves or of others—is one potential solution.

Lies to Maintain Self-Esteem

People with low self-esteem often experience a sense of failure or inferiority because their abilities and accomplishments fall short of their personal expectations for themselves. To use a term coined by Heinz Kohut, the person may feel pressure from the *grandiose self* to achieve remarkable success. Failure to do so (even when the person might be considered successful by usual standards) then results in self-devaluation and guilt. In an effort to regulate self-esteem, the individual may use prevarication in an attempt to close the gap between reality and the grandiose demands. One can see this effect in day-to-day social relationships when ostensibly normal persons embroider the truth, exaggerate, or embellish abilities or accomplishments to appear more successful and admirable. The following are some examples to illustrate how lying supports self-esteem:

▎ A man whose occupational success fell short of his ambitions often reminisced with friends and relatives about his college years when he was a football hero. In fact, he had been a third-string team member who rarely played in a game.

▎ A timid and sexually inexperienced college man boasted of his numerous sexual conquests to his fraternity brothers.

▎ A relatively new medical school department chairman, while at an out-of-town speaking engagement, boasted of his successes in recruiting to his department a large number of new faculty (whose names were not provided), inflating the actual number considerably. Although this man was successful by usual standards, his need for extraordinary accomplishment may have been stimulated by his internal comparisons with his very distinguished and professional brother.

Lies to Create a Sense of Identity

As with the wish-fulfillment lie, the lie told in an effort to bolster self-esteem brings only temporary gratification. The lies must be told repeatedly to increase their credibility. At times, they may take on the character of a personal myth and essentially become part of the memories of the individual involved. For example, the "memories" of combat duty reported by presidential candidate Pat Robertson were not substantiated by his military service record (Edwards 1987). The risk of such lies is, of course, exposure and humiliation. With this type of narcissistic injury, self-esteem may again plunge, and interpersonal relationships may be irretrievably damaged.

A much more pathological and pervasive form of lying and deceit is that which occurs with impostors (see Chapter 8). These individuals may assume various roles, even that of a practicing physician, and live ongoing lies. It has been proposed that these individuals act out their imposture in an attempt to achieve a sense of identity and confidence (Greenacre 1958a, 1958b). In a similar vein, Deutsch (1955) suggested that impostors strive to eliminate friction between an exaggerated ego ideal (the grandiose self) and the devalued, inferior, guilt-ridden part of their egos (their sense of self). She also stated that these impostors behave as if their ego ideals were identical to their sense of self, and they expect everyone else to acknowledge this to be the case. In other words, acceptance of the deceit by others soothes the impostor and reduces the internal conflicts. Thus, the impostor attempts to fool himself or herself that his or her life is not a lie.

Summary

The preceding exploration of the reasons people lie leads to several conclusions.

1. People lie for overtly clear external reasons that will benefit or protect themselves or others. Such lies may have concrete benefit for the individual or for the individual's social network.
2. An individual may lie (deceive) in an effort to regulate self-esteem. This is closely related to efforts to self-deceive, which are moderated primarily through the ego-defense mechanisms.
3. People may lie to others to obtain temporary vicarious gratification (wish-fulfillment lies).
4. Lies, regardless of their content, may protect the sense of an autonomous self and help in differentiating oneself from potentially symbiotic relationships.
5. Lying may serve to attack others, reflecting conscious or unconscious sadistic impulses.
6. The very process of lying and "putting something over" on another person may create a sense of power and superiority; other

people are held in contempt for their inability to detect the lie.

7. Lying is often a reciprocal relationship between the liar and the person to whom the lie is told. An individual may facilitate the process of another person's lying because of the need for self-deceit.

To a large extent the preceding conclusions have a repetitive theme. We lie to ourselves and to others in an effort to support our sense of self-esteem, power, and individuality. We encourage other people to lie to us in order to support our own self-deceit. To reprise Nietzsche, the most common lies are those we tell to ourselves.

Everyone lies to some degree, for the various motives outlined above, but some people have much greater needs for deceit than do others. In the following three chapters, I describe more pervasive forms of lying. In many respects, pathological lying is on a continuum with normal lying; the same issues are involved but to a greater extent.

Chapter 6

Styles of Deception: The Role of Personality

> *Her dramatic, attention-seeking, and histrionic behavior*
> *indeed went to the extent of lying to achieve her aims.*
> *Seeking attention was a way of life to Scarlett, and if*
> *she had to exaggerate, act, or even lie, these acts were*
> *merely tools, used by her with an artisan's skill.*

> —Wells 1976, in reference to Scarlett O'Hara

Different people tell different types of lies for different reasons. This simple statement appears to be a truism. Every person tends to have a characteristic manner in which he or she handles the "truth." This includes not only one's deceptive communications with others but also the characteristic manner of self-deception. Personality is important in determining these patterns of deception and self-deception; conversely, the style of deception is one aspect of personality.

Personality and Lying

Personality is a term used to describe a person's habits or behavior patterns that characterize his or her adjustment to life. These be-

103

haviors and responses include coping styles, ways of relating to other people, moral values, and emotional responses (Fuller and LeRoy 1993). Different forms of stress call for different coping mechanisms, and most people have developed a wide range of intrapsychic and interpersonal techniques in order to survive the perceived and real crises of everyday life. Even so, most people have such characteristic mannerisms and styles of doing things that we can describe them as having unique personalities.

People who have fairly stereotypical behavior and inflexibility in their coping styles, regardless of the form of stress, are often labeled as having personality disorders. Because of this inflexibility, their responses to some forms of stress are often inappropriate. Typically, people with personality disorders see their life problems as caused by others or by misfortune rather than by themselves. The personality disorders constitute one diagnostic category in DSM-IV (American Psychiatric Association 1994), and there are specific diagnostic criteria for 10 different personality disorders.

In a previous work, my colleagues and I identified five specific personality disorders in which lying is a frequent occurrence (Ford et al. 1988). We were not indicating that lying does not occur with other personality disorders or in the absence of personality disorders; rather, we were able to identify deception as a predominant characteristic behavior for these five personalities. In a sense, we can use these categories to identify five specific types of liars.

The antisocial, histrionic, borderline, and narcissistic personality disorders fit into what has been termed the *Cluster B* category of personality disorders in DSM-IV. These disorders have several common traits, and many psychiatrists regard them as variations on a theme. Their differences are determined by exhibited behavior, but the underlying character structures are similar (Kernberg 1975). Obsessive-compulsive personality disorder, the fifth personality disorder discussed below, is placed in *Cluster C,* which also includes the avoidant and dependent personality disorders.

Each of the five personalities described in this chapter is relatively common, and the reader should have no difficulty in recognizing them from experiences of everyday life. However, one caution is that the presence of one or two features does not establish the diagnosis of a personality disorder. Many persons have traits of a personality disorder, but the actual diagnosis is based on a pervasive lifelong pattern of a number of characteristic behaviors. Furthermore, although these are distinct categories in a diagnostic manual, in real life their boundaries tend to blur.

Antisocial Personality Disorder

"He'll charm the pants off you while stealing your wallet"; so said Billy Joe's elementary school principal when Billy Joe was only 11 years old.

Later, when Billy Joe was 29 years old, Sarah found this description to be literally true. She met him while standing in the checkout line of the local supermarket. Billy Joe was handsome in an indescribable fashion, despite irregular facial features. He wore a gold chain visible beneath his open shirt and was carrying a Bible (an affectation that he had discovered helped him sell cars in a small southern town). He was outgoing, friendly, and self-assured; when he asked Sarah for her telephone number, she—somewhat to her surprise—gave it to him. He was different from the type of man to whom she was usually attracted. She continued to be surprised by her subsequent behavior in her relationship with Billy Joe. Sarah rationalized it as "really being in love for the first time" and "learning how to be less inhibited." Friends commented on how she was "blossoming" and was no longer just a mousy, 35-year-old schoolteacher.

Within a relatively short time Billy Joe had moved in with this pillar of the Baptist young adult Sunday school class. Sarah was vaguely troubled, not only because of the moral implications but also because she knew so little about him. When she asked about his past and family, he gave her glib superficial answers. Still, it was obvious that he "adored" her as no man had before, and that was exhilarating. He tended to drink too much, but she was sure that she could control it, perhaps with help from her preacher after they were married.

Billy Joe had proposed marriage early in their relationship but had delayed it with the excuse that he needed to get his financial affairs in order. He had a "new job" at the local Chevrolet dealer selling cars and wanted to be able to "properly support" a wife before marrying her. In the meantime, he borrowed money from Sarah, who helped him cheerfully.

As the months went by and the excuses mounted, Sarah pressed harder to set a wedding date. Finally, Billy Joe "confessed" that he had been previously married in California and that it wasn't completely resolved; the lawyer had to be paid, and some other matters had to be taken care of before the final divorce decree could be obtained. Brokenhearted and tearful, Sarah gave Billy Joe $2,500 to go to California to settle his marital situation. He said that he would be back in 2 weeks, but she never heard from him again.

Months later, when her grief had largely resolved, she took her wounded pride to the local police chief. He ran a computer search and informed her that Billy Joe had served one jail term for breaking and entering and that there were warrants pending in several states for unpaid traffic tickets. Billy Joe's deceit and fraud of Sarah were only one small part of a lifelong pattern.

Billy Joe was the youngest of three children born in a small southern town to a part-time used-car salesman, who was a full-time philanderer and abusive alcoholic. Billy Joe's mother supported the children by working in a shirt factory. When not working, she was preoccupied by her activities in a local fundamentalist church. Billy Joe began engaging in petty theft and shoplifting while still in grade school. He had discovered that he could look someone straight in the eye, say "Sir" or "Ma'am," and get away with almost anything. Once, he was almost caught for breaking a neighbor's window. He blamed it on another child (who was whipped for this transgression) and later bragged to friends about his cleverness.

Billy Joe was bright, verbally skillful, and managed to graduate from high school despite marginal grades and several suspensions for various misbehaviors. He was drafted into the military and had continual conflict with authority figures, and after several brief unauthorized absences, he was given an administrative discharge as "unsuitable for military service."

Billy Joe would receive a diagnosis of antisocial personality disorder from a psychiatrist. Billy Joe's life was characterized by deceit, disregard for the rights of others, instability in work and interpersonal relationships, and repeated brushes with the law.

Persons with antisocial personality disorders (known in the past as constitutional psychopaths or sociopathic personalities) are characterized by their lack of remorse for their misbehavior. They have also been accused of having "cancer of the conscience" or "dry rot

of the superego." It is the very lack of anxiety concerning their behavior that makes them such effective liars. Billy Joe could, as a
child, look straight into the eye of an adult and tell outrageous lies
that were believed. When another child was whipped because of his
lie, he not only felt no guilt but also bragged about his cleverness.
Later, he lied with ease to Sarah about his past and his marital intentions. The emotional and financial repercussions of his lies on
others were of little concern to him, unless they directly affected
him in a negative way.

Pathological lying, deceptions, and manipulations are part of the
core clinical features of the antisocial personality disorder (Hare et
al. 1989; Rogers et al. 1992). The capacity of the sociopathic person
to deceive, cheat, and lie convincingly is described in the classic
work *The Mask of Sanity,* by Hervey Cleckley (1976), and by investigators who have followed him (Hare 1986). The person with an
antisocial personality often has trouble with any type of authority
(e.g., military, legal, and professional) because of difficulty in toler-
ating frustration or delay of gratification. Like small children, they
want what they want when they want it. They have few internal
controls or inhibitions and do not learn from experience. The sociopathic person may be a petty criminal, con artist, or serial killer
(Hare et al. 1989). Many persons with antisocial personalities also
abuse alcohol or other drugs (Cadoret 1986), but it is not necessarily
true that people who abuse substances have antisocial personalities.
Exploitation in interpersonal relationships and sexual promiscuity
are also commonly observed behaviors. Pervasive lying, a prominent
feature of the antisocial personality, is one method that these individuals have learned to get what they want.

Harry (1992a, 1992b) has studied lying in imprisoned criminals.
Not surprisingly, a large proportion of these criminals were sociopathic, and of these, a large proportion had documented pathological
lying. Most of the subjects in the last group, Harry found, continued
to blame others for their crimes or to use a variety of patently flimsy
rationalizations for their behavior and incarceration. It was obvious
that these criminals had not learned from their experience and were
adept at using words to deceive others—and themselves—about
their behavior and its consequences.

Persons with antisocial personality disorder constitute about

2%–3% of the general population; they are more frequently male than female, by a ratio of about four to one. Antisocial personality disorders are more prevalent in persons who live in suburbs than in small towns, and in persons who live in urban areas than in suburban settings (Cadoret 1986). Some researchers believe hysteria (see below) is the female counterpart of the antisocial personality (Guze et al. 1971).

Sociopathy is believed to be caused by an interaction of biological factors and environmental experiences (Cadoret et al. 1990). The role of genetic influence has been repeatedly demonstrated in studies of adopted children. Children, even those who have been adopted and raised by nonsociopathic parents, whose biological parent was sociopathic have an increased risk of becoming sociopathic personalities themselves. Environmental experiences that are important in the genesis of sociopathy include having been raised in a chaotic or inconsistent home that had disregard for societal values or that was influenced by alcoholism.

One research study suggested that persistent and extreme childhood lying is an important predictor of adult antisocial behavior and that lying may be a fundamental underpinning of other antisocial behaviors (Hare et al. 1989). That certainly seemed to be the case with Billy Joe, who used lying effectively as a child to support other misbehavior.

When genetic causes are suggested for apparently deviant behavior, one must ask why they exist. Why, in the course of evolution and the "survival of the fittest," should a characteristic or grouping of characteristics that is not apparently adaptive persist through hundreds of generations rather than being gradually eliminated through differential reproduction? One troubling explanation could be that antisocial behavior is, in fact, adaptive: "Crime does pay!" (see Chapter 13.) Another possible explanation is that antisocial behavior was adaptive during human evolution before civilization and that we are now looking at atavistic remnants of characteristics that were an effective means of survival thousands of years ago.

Yet another fascinating hypothesis for explaining the persistence of antisocial personality features incorporates the use of deceit into the theory of parental investment. Parental investment is a concept proffered by Robert Trivers (1985) at the University of California,

Santa Cruz. He suggests that parents who invest in the care of their offspring will, as a result, have a higher percentage of offspring who reach maturity (and become reproductive) than those parents who put fewer of their resources into parenting. However, if the number of offspring of low-investment parents is sufficiently greater than that of high-investment parents, then the absolute number of offspring who reach reproductive age may exceed that of the high-investment parents (e.g., 60% of five is greater than 80% of three). That is, even though more children of high-investment parents may reach maturity, there may be more children of low-investment parents to begin with, so those traits would not be eliminated. Both reproductive strategies (low-investment and high-investment) may, at different times in human history, be adaptive.

What is the relation of this theory to lying? Two basic features of the antisocial personality are lying and promiscuity. In Chapter 3, which contains a discussion of deceit in lower species, I observed that deceit (lying) is commonly used to increase sexual opportunities. Similar observations are frequently made about people with an antisocial personality such as Billy Joe (Cleckley 1976; Hare 1986). Thus, these two characteristics cluster together in a way that suggests the possibility of increased reproduction rates despite lower parental investment.

Dysfunction in language has also been proposed as an underlying biological factor that relates deceit to the antisocial personality. Research by Hare and colleagues (1989) has indicated that sociopathic persons may have a poor integration of the factual and emotional components of speech. Thus, words do not have the same emotional coloring for sociopaths that they do for nonsociopathic persons. This can lead to fewer constraints in the use of language and "for the psychopath, lying is just a matter of moving words around" (p. 34). This deficiency of emotional connotation of words and language may cause a lack of empathy with others, who are regarded as objects to be manipulated. Deceit is the prerequisite of manipulation.

It has also been proposed that the autonomic nervous system of sociopaths differs from that of healthy people. Sociopaths have a decreased capacity to develop conditioned autonomic nervous system response (e.g., sweating, increased heart rate, and muscular tension) to adverse stimuli (Lykken 1957; Patrick 1994). As a consequence, they often exhibit less fear of dangerous situations and may also not have pronounced response to internal stimuli such as guilt. One can theorize that the lack of these uncomfortable bodily sensations in response to certain stimuli is one reason they do not learn from experience and why they can lie so convincingly. Because their lies are not associated with guilt, there are fewer bodily symptoms to betray the deceit ("leakage," see Chapter 10) to the target of the lie. Similarly, because of these decreased autonomic responses, they may find it easier to fool the lie detector (polygraph).

Yet another characteristic of persons with antisocial personality disorder is a significantly increased rate of frontal-lobe dysfunction and other forms of cognitive impairment compared with that of healthy persons (Burgess 1992; Gorenstein 1982). These findings were discussed in Chapter 3.

Histrionic Personality Disorder

"Did you remember to return the videos?" asked Rick.

"Sure, honey," Cindy lied skillfully and then embroidered her story: "Boy, was it ever busy! I had to wait in line for 10 minutes."

"Good, I hate paying for those extra days," replied Rick.

Later, when Rick went out to Cindy's car to look for his sweater, he found the videotapes on the front seat. He returned to the apartment in a rage, stating that he was sick and tired of being lied to. He then recounted the episode the previous week when she had assured him that she had plenty of money in her account to pay for a new dress she had bought, only to ask him for money to cover a bounced check a few days later.

As usual, Cindy was penitent; she cried and said that she was only trying to protect him from getting angry about unimportant details. After all, she had meant to return the tapes but had forgotten; she would have put them in the drop box before the store opened in the morning. And she had only bought the new dress because she knew Rick would like it. To demonstrate her true love for Rick, Cindy became very affectionate and sexually provocative. As usual, Rick forgave her.

At the time of this altercation, Rick and Cindy had been married for 9 months. Their marriage had been a series of peaks and valleys with intense fights (often about Cindy's lies or disregard for financial matters) and equally torrid reconciliations. Their first major fight had occurred shortly after the wedding, when Rick learned that Cindy had "forgotten" to tell him that she owed several thousand dollars on her credit cards, and Rick's budget projections were therefore invalid. Cindy would often spend money on a whim and then attempt to keep her purchases a secret or try to spring them on Rick when he was in a good mood. Because of this pattern, Rick had become progressively more suspicious and had started to check on her in various ways.

Because Cindy worked as a receptionist for a major corporation and was expected to dress attractively, she could use this excuse for some of her purchases. In fact, she had met Rick, an accountant, when he visited the company for the annual audit. He liked her attractiveness, her cheery smile, and her good humor. Cindy was a contrast to the more serious woman he had been seeing; she brought excitement to his life. She found his solid dependability and stability a welcome change from the more flighty men she had been dating.

Cindy was the youngest of three children born to the family of a career Marine Corps officer who was often away from home. She romanticized her father, seeing him as a hero serving his country. He was very affectionate with Cindy, who was his favorite child, and would bring her expensive gifts from foreign countries. In fact, Cindy believed that her father preferred her to her more emotionally distant mother who complained too much about his heavy drinking.

Several traumatic events occurred in Cindy's developmental years. She was a fervent believer in Santa Claus (encouraged by her parents and older siblings) and was devastated to learn from first-grade classmates that he was only a myth. She also learned, during a parental fight in her teenage years, that her mother had been previously married (a family secret) and that her father was having an affair with another woman. Shortly thereafter, Cindy became sexually active and indiscriminately promiscuous; this behavior resulted in a pregnancy and subsequent abortion. Her sexual behavior caused great dismay to her parents, who were devout fundamentalist Protestants and could not understand why Cindy was not following the teachings of their church.

Cindy was an average student who performed below her capabilities in school. She became easily bored and picked up—and dropped—one interest after another. Because she wasn't interested in studying, she dropped out of college after one semester and became a secretary. However, this was also boring. She took a job as a receptionist, with a pay cut, because she found it more fun to meet people, especially the men who visited the company. When Cindy met Rick, she portrayed her family, adolescence, and college experiences with a glowing "all-American" description. She told him that she was a college graduate and had been a cheerleader. The more sordid details of her life, which would eventually emerge, were glossed over with glib fabrications.

Divorce from Rick was inevitable, and Cindy is now "working" on her third husband, but this marriage is also shaky. She is confused about why both Rick and her second husband were so angry and why they do not want even minimal contact with her. Rick had finally filed for divorce after he learned of a series of purchases that Cindy had made (but denied) that almost required the couple to file for bankruptcy. Feeling depressed after her second divorce, Cindy sought help in psychotherapy but gave it up after several sessions. She complained that she often felt worse rather than feeling better, as she had hoped, because the therapist made her think about things that she was trying to forget.

Similar to the lies told by Billy Joe, Cindy's lies were convincing. She often elaborated on the basic lie to make it appear more believable. She would frequently lie even when it served little purpose, yet she did not feel particularly guilty about it. To the contrary, she rationalized that she was only trying to keep people from becoming upset. She herself easily forgot unpleasant things very quickly and could not understand why others became upset at her when she meant so well. Her style was to flatter people (usually insincerely) so frequently that it was second nature and it really never even entered her consciousness.

Cindy wanted people to like her and, somewhat childlike, she attempted to avoid unpleasantness or responsibility. She tended to see things in an emotional manner and could not be bothered by exact details (such as her bank account balance).

Cindy can be described as having a histrionic personality style. An older, but still frequently used, term is *hysteria.* Hysteria is a word dating to antiquity that has been used to describe a variety of psychiatric phenomena, including a personality style, medically unexplained physical symptoms, or a specified psychoanalytic construct (Chodoff and Lyons 1958). Here, hysteria refers to personality style and, in accordance with common usage, will be more or less synonymous with the histrionic personality disorder. Hysteria can be described as a continuum. Relatively normal persons with hysterical personality traits who are dramatic and use repression represent one pole. At the other extreme are those persons who meet the diagnostic criteria for histrionic personality disorder. They demonstrate a considerably greater degree of psychopathology and share many characteristics of the borderline personality disorder (see below). (For a more detailed exposition of this subject, refer to Chodoff 1974; Easser and Lesser 1965; or Kernberg 1975, 1985a.)

During the past two to three decades disagreement has been ongoing as to the cause of histrionic (hysterical) personality traits. Psychoanalysts have traditionally viewed hysterical traits as the result of incompletely resolved psychological issues related to the oedipal period of development. For example, a girl may have incompletely resolved her competitive feelings with her mother and therefore failed to establish a healthy identification with her mother and a firm self-identity as a woman. The primary psychological mechanism used by the person with histrionic personality disorder is generally repression, although displacement, dissociation, and acting out are also prominent. In the more severe disorder, "splitting" (described below) becomes a more predominant ego mechanism (Kernberg 1985a).

In contrast to the psychoanalysts, biologically oriented psychiatrists believe that hysterical personality traits are determined more by hereditary factors and are closely related to the antisocial personality features. Genetic studies have demonstrated that the same families that tend to produce sons with antisocial personalities also tend to produce daughters with hysterical personalities. Thus, it has been suggested that the two disorders share a common etiology but that expressed personality features are due to gender and cultural expectations of behavior (Guze et al. 1971).

Regardless of which theory may be more accurate (the biological view of behavior is currently in ascendancy), there is little doubt that, similar to the antisocial personality, issues related to deceit and sexual behavior are frequently described in the person with a histrionic personality. The richest of these descriptions comes from psychoanalysts who have worked closely with these persons in psychotherapy. Dr. Marc Hollender (1971), a distinguished psychiatrist and scholar of hysteria, described these people as most likely to be dishonest when seeking attention or feeling threatened by rejection. He stated that for histrionic women, the line between wishing and reality is easily blurred. They are suggestible and gullible, and "affective truth" (if it feels right, it must be true) often overrides facts or logic. Hollender went on to describe these women as very self-centered, wishing to be entertained, and extremely demanding. They are also characterized by a low tolerance for frustration. Women with histrionic personalities are often strikingly seductive when relating to men, despite the fact that they are frequently sexually dysfunctional; their sexuality is often used to manipulate men. To quote Hollender, "Early marriage and a high incidence of divorce are parts of the pattern. So, too, are many premarital and extramarital affairs" (p. 19).

Seymour Halleck, another eminent psychiatrist, has also studied hysteria, and his phenomenological descriptions of hysterical personality traits also sound similar to descriptions of sociopathy. "The hysteric personality's demanding nature, histrionics, and dishonesty should be viewed as purposeful actions designed to structure the interpersonal situation so that she can manipulate the responses of others in a manner which assures their continued interest and affection" (Halleck 1967, p. 750). Halleck also detailed the dishonesty of women with histrionic personalities in their interpersonal relationships and with their therapists when they enter psychiatric treatment. He noted the close relation with antisocial behavior and reported that institutionalized female delinquents, when deprived of access to antisocial behavior, quickly turn to hysterical behavior as an adaptive device. This behavior is characterized by a demanding nature, dependency, histrionics, dishonesty, and a preoccupation with sexuality.

In their description of how persons with histrionic personality behave in psychiatric interviews, MacKinnon and Michels (1971) described dramatization and exaggeration that can proceed to overt confabulation (fabrication). These authors commented that "the patient exaggerates in order to dramatize a viewpoint and is unconcerned about rigid adherence to truth if a distortion will better accomplish the drama" (p. 112). MacKinnon and Michels also noted that these persons are often sexually promiscuous. As noted above, these persons may dress provocatively and draw attention to themselves. This characteristic might be viewed in a basic biological sense as using "lures" to attract sexual partners (see Chapter 3).

As noted above, persons with a histrionic personality disorder are often superficially charming and seductive. They are constantly seeking attention by their dress or dramatic mannerisms. They are emotional rather than intellectual and, often in a childish manner, expect others to care for them. They often report details about their lives, including their medical histories, in a dramatic, imprecise manner with more attention to performance than to accuracy. For example, instead of saying that she had had a simple appendectomy, Cindy would dramatically tell how she was saved just in the nick of time before her appendix ruptured.

Hysteria is often regarded as a woman's disease, but it is by no means exclusive to women; many men have hysteria. Males who have histrionic tendencies may also have antisocial traits and may thus be more frequently labeled as antisocial personalities. As noted above, antisocial and histrionic personality are closely related to each other, and the expression of certain personality features may largely be a matter of gender. Persons with histrionic personality usually have at least some antisocial traits; Cindy was not especially guilty about either her lying or her financial irresponsibility.

Persons with histrionic personalities are renowned for their skills in lying, but their prevarication does not usually have the malignant quality that is evident in the lying of persons with antisocial personality. More frequently, it is to create a dramatic effect, to avoid unpleasantness, or to get people to like them (the ingratiating lie). However, their deceit ultimately takes its toll. The superficiality of these people, their lack of genuine feelings beneath the surface storm of emotion, and the anger engendered in others from being repeatedly deceived (even in minor ways) drive other people away and makes true intimacy difficult, if not impossible.

Persons with hysteria are exceptionally skilled at self-deception.

These persons exclude unpleasant thoughts (or facts) from consciousness by using repression, and hide the true nature of their life and behavior from themselves by using dissociation, displacement, and projection.

Borderline Personality Disorder

"What do you mean you're not pregnant?!" Bob screamed at Barbara.

"Well, I thought I was. Maybe I had a miscarriage," responded a somewhat contrite, but sullenly defiant, Barbara.

It was 3 weeks after the wedding, and Barbara had been unsuccessful in hiding from Bob the fact that she was having a normal menstrual period. For the preceding month, she had skillfully avoided this confrontation and had even feigned nausea and fatigue on a daily basis. Six weeks previously, during one of their many quarrels, Bob had indicated that it was time to end their tumultuous relationship. In response, Barbara made a tearful "confession" that she was pregnant but indicated that because of her love for Bob she would carry the baby to term regardless of what he wanted to do. Beset with feelings of guilt and obligation, Bob responded with an offer of marriage. Whirlwind plans for a small, formal wedding had followed.

At the time of her marriage, Barbara was 29 years old, acutely aware of her age and her increasing tendency to gain weight easily. Her relationships with men had a repetitive quality to them. They typically had begun with intense infatuation on the part of Barbara. She would see each new man in her life as the person who would be able to love and support her. As each relationship progressed, she would make increasing demands until the man would resist. Barbara would then angrily attack him for being self-centered and not caring enough about her. After several such fights the relationship would inevitably end, and Barbara would bitterly complain to all who would listen about having once again been abused.

On one occasion, after a breakup with a lover, Barbara made a dramatic suicide gesture with an overdose of Valium, a medication that she periodically abused. She was hospitalized in a psychiatric unit for 3 days and was then released. Barbara was in and out of psychotherapy several times. Each period of therapy was with a different psychiatrist, one of whom refused to see her again after she verbally abused him during a 3:00 A.M. telephone call while she was intoxicated.

Barbara's pattern of lying was first noted at an early age, when she fabricated stories to schoolmates about her home life. These "fantastic" tales included descriptions of a rich uncle who would pick her up in his black Cadillac and take her to exciting places, such as Disneyland. These stories were in stark contrast to the real nature of Barbara's life. In truth, she lived a drab, unhappy existence. Her father was a passive furniture salesman who was perpetually bitter that he was repeatedly passed over for promotion to assistant manager. His only excursions from his passive role occurred when he would drink to excess, become belligerent, and verbally (and occasionally physically) abuse his wife and Barbara. Barbara's mother never stopped complaining—about her husband, Barbara, the rabbi, or life in general. She would periodically remind Barbara that "it is lucky for you that abortion used to be illegal."

As she grew older, Barbara became increasingly envious of other girls who had more expensive clothes or whose families she regarded as happier. At times, the envy took on a malignant quality, and she would invent or pass along malicious rumors about her classmates.

She graduated from high school and then nursing school. She had difficulty maintaining jobs for lengthy periods but, because of the nursing shortage, rarely had difficulty in finding new positions. She often made snide and inaccurate comments about other nurses or the attending physicians. On one occasion she was fired because she came to work intoxicated on Valium.

Seven years after their marriage (which was marked by her angry accusations, Bob's depressed withdrawal, and no children), Bob developed renal failure associated with chronic hypertension. Barbara was disgusted by his illness and his need for help with home renal dialysis. She complained that he was an inadequate husband and filed for divorce on the basis of incompatibility.

Almost everyone knows someone like Barbara. Such people are unhappy, unpleasant troublemakers who go through life with a marginal level of adjustment. Diagnostically, they have borderline personality disorder, a misnomer from the past when the disorder was thought to be on the borderline of schizophrenia. However, current etiological concepts place this personality disorder closer to the mood disorders and impulse control disorders (Silverman et al. 1991; Soloff et al. 1991). Another biological characteristic, demonstrated in recent research, is that these persons usually have decreased levels of serotonin (a major neurotransmitter) in their brains. Reduced brain serotonin has been shown to be related to impulsiveness (Stein et al. 1993). Yet another biological feature is a high frequency of subtle cognitive dysfunction (see Chapter 3).

Regardless of etiological considerations, the background and behavior of the person with borderline personality characteristics have a familiar pattern. These people typically come from "dysfunctional" families that had a chaotic undercurrent, even when the family appeared relatively normal to outsiders. Parental alcoholism or drug abuse has been frequently observed, and sexual or physical abuse is also frequently reported (G. R. Brown and Anderson 1991; Herman et al. 1989).

The behavior of the borderline person is often characterized by impulsive behavior, including self-destructive acts. There may be problems with alcohol, drugs, shopping sprees, or promiscuity (American Psychiatric Association 1994). Moods are intense and may change abruptly. Relationships are tenuous, with the other person often initially idealized and later devalued. Envy and overtly jealous behavior are frequently seen, and these people may construct elaborate fantasies of a wish-fulfilling nature that they communicate to others as fact. Other common fabrications are about how they have suffered or been abused in the past. For example, the lie of one woman with borderline personality disorder included the story that she had been captured and tortured (Ford 1973). Lies or misrepresentations concerning sexual abuse and rape may also occur (M. D. Feldman et al. 1994). There is an undercurrent of pervasive anger interrupted only by periodic eruptions of overt rage.

The lies of the person with borderline personality disorder reflect several features of the underlying characteristics of the disorder. These persons have poor impulse control; words may be said without the degree of reflection used by most people. Such communication may be more fantasy than fact. The borderline person may also use fantasy as a way of soothing himself or herself, and the fantasy becomes more real if it is communicated to another person who responds to it as if it were true. Through the mechanism of

pseudologia fantastica, the borderline person may construct fantasies that are communicated to others as fact. As a child, Barbara used
this mechanism to create a fantasy about a rich and kindly uncle,
both to soothe herself in reference to her bleak reality and to make
her feel more important to her friends.

The person with borderline personality disorder is usually an
angry, vengeful person who uses lies as weapons. For example, a
spurned woman may accuse her former lover of rape and actually
file charges against him (S. Snyder 1986). Barbara maliciously
spread false rumors about people toward whom she felt jealousy. Lies
may be used to manipulate other people with little consideration for
their needs or feelings. This is illustrated by Barbara's lie about pregnancy to maintain her relationship with Bob.

Persons with borderline personality disorder use several primitive psychological mechanisms for self-deception. Prominent is the
use of *splitting*. This term describes two different types of behavior,
both characteristic of the disorder. Interpersonally, splitting refers
to the way in which people with borderline disorder play people
against each other; this is often accomplished by lies and rumors.
For example, a woman with a drug abuse problem tried to create
dissension between two of her physicians who were attempting to
coordinate prescriptions for her. She told Doctor A that Doctor B
had said Doctor A was not up-to-date in his knowledge of pharma-
cology. This manipulative behavior often places the perpetrator at
the center of attention and also creates a (false) sense of control and
power. Splitting is also an intrapsychic mechanism. It is truly a form
of self-deception because various ideas and feelings are "split" apart
from one another and poorly integrated. Thus, the many internally
contradictory aspects of these people's inner lives are kept separate
to reduce psychological discomfort. For example, depending on the
circumstances, a person involved with someone who has borderline
personality disorder may at different times be viewed as "all good"
or "all bad." This mechanism facilitates the rapid switches in interpersonal relationships in which a person may be idealized and then
devalued.

People with borderline features also typically use projection, dissociation, and acting out as ego-defense mechanisms to perpetuate
their self-deception (see Chapter 2). Barbara characteristically used

splitting (idealizing and devaluing Bob), projection (claiming Bob could not meet her needs when she was the one who could not care for him), and acting out (abusing habituating medications) as methods to deal with her psychological pain.

Of all the people whom psychiatrists treat, persons with borderline personality disorder are among the most difficult. They relate to their therapists with the various behaviors described above and usually distort, conceal, or lie about aspects of their personal lives, both past and present. When they start treatment, they tend to idealize the therapist, but later they are prone to angry devaluation. They are manipulative and often claim to others that the therapist said something that, in fact, was not communicated. They may also threaten, or execute, suicidal or other self-destructive behaviors. If sufficiently angry, borderline persons may file malicious malpractice suits or make false allegations about their therapists (or other) physicians) to ethics committees or medical licensing boards (M. D. Feldman and Ford 1994).

Narcissistic Personality Disorder

At the annual company Christmas party, Marshall moved somewhat awkwardly from one small group of junior corporate officers to another. He talked rapidly and loudly, often interrupting others and boasting of his successes during the past year. "Sales have been the highest in two decades." "I have recruited the best district managers in the country." "My new sales campaign has taken the South by storm." Interspersed were periodic comments about "my days at the Harvard School of Business" and allusions to his father, who was president of another major corporation. Ruth, Marshall's wife, followed him to skillfully attempt to smooth the wake of ruffled feathers left by Marshall. By smiling, flattering, and asking personal questions about work and home, she was to a large extent successful. When Marshall joined a group of more senior corporate officers, he suddenly became quieter and more deferential as he flattered them and then moved on.

Later that night on their way home from the party, an irritated Ruth confronted Marshall: "I am sick and tired of your telling everyone how great you are. You know damn well that it was Bosworth, whom you fired, who was responsible for the southern advertising campaign. And where the hell do you get off on Harvard Business School? You only attended one weekend seminar there!"

In truth, Marshall's position with the company was shaky because of poor interpersonal skills and his limited capacity to follow through on his grandiose projects. He continued to maintain his position largely because of his superiors' reluctance to fire him because of his well-known family connections.

Marshall had met Ruth in his mid-20s, during his tenure as an active-duty naval officer. He was dashing in his dress blues, which he wore (unnecessarily) to a family cocktail party. Ruth, who was rather mousy in appearance, was "taken" by this handsome young officer who talked grandly of his business prospects when he completed his naval service. She was also impressed by Marshall's rather pointed references to his influential family. In turn, Marshall was impressed by the fact that Ruth was impressed by him, and he asked her for a date.

Because Ruth was socially astute and ambitious and knew that her other prospects were not any better, she skillfully flattered Marshall throughout their courtship. Later, after they were married, Ruth discovered that her "prize catch" was less desirable than she had originally judged. He was insecure, sensitive to criticism, vain, self-preoccupied, and "used her" rather than appreciated her help and her own qualities. Perhaps most importantly for her, Marshall seemed unable to function effectively in the role of the aggressive young businessman that he had projected. He did not follow through on his grandiose plans, and Ruth learned that he had exaggerated his past accomplishments. His insensitivity to the feelings of others tended to cause interpersonal strife, leaving him alienated. Yet, despite this, Ruth regarded herself as "in it for the long haul" and learned not only how to keep shoring up Marshall's shaky self-esteem but also to put her own social skills to work in order to help him at his job.

Although Marshall was fairly oblivious at a conscious level to Ruth's help, he remained loyal to her and, with her quiet assistance, managed to continue functioning at a marginal level. Only on occasion, such as after the Christmas party, would she lose her temper.

Marshall was the second son born to the chief executive of a relatively small but well-known industrial manufacturer. The father was preoccupied with his business, and when he had spare time, he tended to spend it with Marshall's older brother, who was more athletic and (in Marshall's opinion) less intelligent. Marshall's mother was a closet alcoholic who would be periodically absent from the home traveling (or in an alcoholism treatment program). Marshall's child care needs were met by the housekeeper, and he did receive some maternal warmth from a woman in the neighborhood whose children were approximately his age. He missed his mother, idealized his father, and envied his brother. He constructed various fantasies in which he would beat his brother in tennis or golf and rise to such a position in the business world that his father would see him as the powerful person he really was.

Despite these ambitious goals and his high intelligence, Marshall seemed unable to perform at a superior level. He would quickly become bored with various activities and move on to something else before he had mastered them. He attended a well-known (but second-rate) college and with the quiet help of family was able to get into the "right" fraternity and later obtain a desirable navy assignment.

Marshall continued in his job, resenting that he had not been promoted and continuing to have fantasies of becoming a powerful figure in industry. His exaggerations and misrepresentations of his abilities quietly made him the butt of many jokes of those who worked with him. His superiors decided that firing him (because of his family connections) might cause more problems than it would solve. Ruth, the mother of three children and loyal to the end, regarded Marshall as her fourth child. Fortunately, a trust fund that began paying income to Marshall when he reached age 35 years kept the family financially comfortable.

Marshall's pattern of behavior fits into the general category of a narcissistic personality disorder. The degree of his dysfunction was not severe, particularly with the support of Ruth, but he certainly performed at a significantly lower level than he perceived. He used exaggerations, half-truths, and even blatant lies to present himself to others as a highly confident and competent businessman. Perhaps more important, he used these prevarications to shield the truth of his limitations from himself.

The current psychoanalytic interpretation of narcissism is that, despite the apparent grandiosity and arrogant self-confidence, these people have low self-esteem (Kernberg 1985b). Their difficulties with regulating self-esteem make them sensitive to failures and slights (often imagined), to which they often react with depression or anger. Furthermore, they are so preoccupied with themselves that they feel entitled to special consideration. They are usually insensitive to the needs of others whom, as a consequence, they often exploit.

Explanations of the low self-esteem of narcissistic individuals largely revolve around early childhood experiences. Children may become self-centered as a result of having too little empathic attention from parents, even though they may have been indulged with many material gifts.

Narcissistic individuals tend to see the world only from their own perspective and are thus prone to lying. These lies are often fueled not so much by sociopathic motives as by the need to perceive and define the world according to their own internal states. At times, when they are feeling powerless, they may lie for the thrilling sensation of putting something over on another person (Bursten 1972).

Many features of narcissistic personality traits were found in the entrepreneurs described by Person (1986). Entrepreneurs manipulate others and are distinguished by boldness, impulse to gamble, and lack of guilty restraint. Narcissistic personality features have been noted in compulsive gamblers who also are prone to self-deception and lying (Hayano 1988; Pyles 1989).

Many observers believe that the incidence of narcissism seems to be increasing. Many putative causes have been blamed, but few hard data exist. Among the proposed etiologies are rapid social change and the societal breakdown of the traditional family unit (Kernberg 1985b). Divorce and blended families are now more frequent, and most mothers work outside the home. Also, cultural changes have been characterized as creating the "me-generation," summarized in the self-oriented concept that "you only go around once." Furthermore, "success" has been increasingly measured by career achievement and the possession of certain material possessions. Advertisers feed this mentality; for example, implying that the purchase of a certain automobile means that "you have arrived."

Descriptions of many politicians (see Chapter 1) appear to be consistent with narcissistic issues. Obtaining power and prestige in the political arena may be a method of attempting to boost an underlying feeling of low self-esteem. The narcissistic person often has poor reality testing; the outside world is perceived in very personal terms, and the internal world is contaminated with grandiosity. Of note, Kernberg (1980) has observed that in times of stress, people may turn toward and look for narcissistic leaders. We should not be surprised by the "lies" of these politicians. They and their constituents are involved in mutual self-deception. The politician says what others want to hear or describes how things should be; neither half of the dyad wants to know the truth.

The relation of narcissism to deceit can be readily observed in everyday life. Narcissistic individuals aspire to power (see Chapter 5) and frequently hold positions of authority. Fueled by their need for self-importance and the need to maintain self-esteem, persons with narcissistic personalities seek and obtain positions of authority and leadership (Kernberg 1980).

Kets de Vries and Miller (1985) described three types of narcissistic personality and the effects of these personality types on their functions in leadership roles. These three types are the reactive narcissist, the self-deceptive narcissist, and the constructive narcissist. The last category reflects a degree of healthy narcissism that often promotes good leadership, but the former two are often problematic. *Reactive narcissists,* who experienced rejecting and unresponsive parenting, are often ruthless in their use of power. They tolerate no disagreement and crush dissension. Their distorted reality (including their self-deceptions and overt lies) must be accepted by underlings if the latter wish to survive in the organization. *Self-deceptive narcissists,* who as children were led by parents to believe that they were lovable and perfect, are often manipulative leaders. Such persons frequently have interpersonal difficulties because of their emotional superficiality and lack of genuine empathy for others. *Constructive narcissists* are ambitious, manipulative, and occasionally opportunistic. They generally get along well with subordinates because they have self-confidence, adaptability, humor, and the capacity to recognize the strengths and needs of other persons. As a result, they are often able to energize subordinates and achieve genuine accomplishments.

Horowitz and Arthur (1988) have described the various effects that narcissistic leaders may have on organizations. They observed that when the self-esteem of a narcissistic person is threatened, he

or she may, in response to narcissistic injury, react with sadistic behaviors. The resulting tension can, in its milder forms, result in
increased self-deception by group members; they will distort their
own views of reality to placate the leader. When the tension becomes
unbearable, "The group processes, in reaction to rages of the leader,
can worsen the situation, leading to ruination, blood baths, or mu-
tiny" (Horowitz and Arthur 1988, p. 141).

Narcissistic persons can be identified in any organization by
their glib manipulativeness and sense of self-importance. A current
"buzzword" for grandiosity is "vision." A person may be recruited
for a position of responsibility and authority on the basis of "vision"
and deceitful promises or misstatements of facts. When the "vision"
fails to materialize or personnel become angry at broken promises,
the narcissistic person turns to comfortable rationalizations. He or
she may say that circumstances have changed, that he or she has
been misunderstood, or that he or she has been deceived and was
only doing the best possible under adverse circumstances.

One may question the relation of narcissism to sociopathy. Both
disorders are characterized by a lack of empathy for others, a deficiency of apparent guilt, and deceitful behavior. A major difference
is that the narcissistic person, because of his or her need for admiration or power, may be able to single-mindedly pursue and achieve
set goals. In contrast, the sociopathic person's inability to delay
gratification and impulsive behavior are frequently self-defeating
and prevent successful attainment of goals.

Obsessive-Compulsive Personality Disorder

Brooks carefully stopped by the library for a minute or two on his
way home from his psychotherapy hour. Thus, when his wife, Mary
Jo, asked the inevitable questions about why he was late, he could
"truthfully" answer that he had been at the library.

For 2 years Brooks had kept from Mary Jo the secret that he was
seeing a psychotherapist. Not surprisingly, one of the topics of his
therapy was the conflicted relationship with his wife, whom he regarded as both controlling and critical. He had expressed the opinion that if he were to tell her that he was seeing a therapist, she
would put a stop to it. Brooks had also become skillful at "stealing

hours" for himself away from work by providing senior members of his law firm with plausible "truthful" (but incomplete) explanations of his absences.

Despite this appearance of passivity, Brooks was actually a successful young attorney who had been targeted for partnership within the next 2–3 years by his prestigious law firm. He was recognized for his meticulous work, particularly in drawing up contracts. The only major complaint lodged against him by senior partners in the firm was his tendency to procrastinate.

Brooks prided himself on his reliability and honesty. He rationalized his tendency to keep secrets and provide selected information as a right to privacy. He would have been offended if he were ever called a liar.

Brooks was an only child raised in the rural South. His father was a laconic man whose parents had lost their farm during the depression. The father's philosophy and few words seemed to revolve around "time is money" and "idle hands are the devil's playground." On a day-to-day basis, his father made every effort to control Brooks's activities, as well as those of his passive, frightened, and chronically ill wife.

To evade his father's insistence that he either do farm chores or study, Brooks developed two strategies. One was to prolong the school day (he was an excellent student) as long as possible through extracurricular activities; the other was to read paperback novels while ostensibly studying. Freedom from his father was finally obtained when Brooks was accepted to a prestigious southern university and his father reluctantly agreed to pay for his college education. A variety of "necessary" summer courses and other programs prevented Brooks from returning home again, except briefly for the holidays. While in law school, Brooks met Mary Jo at his church; she was an attractive, assertive woman who progressively took the initiative in their relationship. Not knowing exactly how it happened, Brooks found himself engaged, married, and the father of a daughter.

Mary Jo and Brooks fought about many issues. She regarded him as stubborn, "stingy," and too preoccupied with his religious beliefs. Furthermore, the house was in continuous disarray because he was a "pack rat" and was unable to throw anything away.

Brooks was in psychotherapy for years. He continued to do satisfactory, but not spectacular, work in the area of contracts and was finally made a partner in his law firm. Mary Jo ultimately learned that he was seeing a psychiatrist and, as Brooks predicted, put an end to his psychotherapy. Brooks responded by having a pathetically furtive affair with one of the paralegals in his office. Mary Jo also learned about the affair and put an end to that as well. Interestingly, she was less upset by the affair than by the psychotherapy. At the time of last contact (a telephone call) Brooks was (secretly) receiving religious instruction and considering conversion from his Southern Baptist roots to the Roman Catholic faith.

One might question the inclusion of Brooks's story into a grouping of liars. His lies seem fairly benign. In fact, he lied to his wife not to cover up a sexual liaison but because he was engaged in psychotherapy. In many respects, Brooks's lies were lies of omission rather than lies of commission. That is, he created a false impression by conveying only part of the truth. This type of deceit is closely associated with keeping secrets. Throughout his life, Brooks had learned (and practiced) the art of maintaining a private life, little known to those closest to him.

From a psychiatric diagnostic viewpoint, Brooks had both obsessive-compulsive and passive-aggressive personality features, a common combination. As a child, his life had been ruled by his controlling father, and he developed techniques to maintain his sense of separateness and as much control over his life as possible. Despite the superficial illogic, Brooks had drifted into a relationship with a woman who had many of the characteristics of his father. Such behavior can be explained by a variety of psychodynamic explanations, possibly including one or more of the following: 1) he was playing a familiar, and therefore comfortable, role; 2) his passiveness kept him from relationships in which he would have had to be more assertive; or 3) he was engaging in a repetition compulsion—a compulsion that occurs when a person repeatedly seeks out a conflictive situation with the unconscious goal of mastering previous psychic trauma (Stoller 1976).

Regardless of why Brooks found himself in such a situation, his pattern of behavior is easily identified. He considered all authority figures, including his superiors at work and his wife, as controlling and intrusive; therefore, he had to maintain secrets, lie, or otherwise mislead them in order to maintain his autonomy. The results of this type of behavior are not particularly malignant, especially when compared with the wide spectrum of human misconduct. Brooks's deceit was not of the same magnitude as the lies told by Barbara or Billy Joe. The major loser was Brooks himself. His secretiveness prevented intimacy and left him a lonely person unable to share his emotions, fears, and joys with others. Constricted, inhibited, and inefficient, he went through life as if the brakes were always partially applied.

The core psychological issue for the obsessive personality is the inner conflict between obedience and defiance (MacKinnon and Michels 1971). This conflict, which emerges in control issues with other persons, often takes on (psychologically speaking) a "life-or-death" importance, even in regard to minor matters. Persons with obsessive-compulsive personality features tend toward perfectionism and rigid behavior. They are often preoccupied with money, time, cleanliness, and issues of right or wrong. Because of their preoccupation with small details, they are often unable to grasp the larger context of a situation (the "big picture"). Their rigidity is also shown by their emotional responses, which are constricted and lack warmth or tenderness. This rigidity includes the area of sexuality, in which they are often inhibited.

Obsessive-compulsive persons frequently report that their childhoods were dominated by other family members who displayed similar traits. Parents were often more mechanical than affectionate and—because of their own rigidity—were very controlling. As a child, the obsessive-compulsive person often develops passive-aggressive behaviors, such as procrastination, indecisiveness, or stubbornness as ways of coping (and rebelling) with the parent's rigidity and control. Both secrecy and lying to protect secrets have been recognized as a part of obsessive psychopathology (Dickes 1968).

Within limited circumstances (e.g., functioning as a neurosurgeon or as an accountant), obsessive-compulsive people can be highly effective. They do, however, tend to withhold their emotions, maintain secrets, and have fairly sterile relationships with other persons.

As noted, obsessive-compulsive persons can be very deceptive.

Although they rationalize this by taking (inappropriate) pride in their honesty and truthfulness, they provide only part of the truth, thereby creating misperceptions. This type of deception can be very useful in the practice of law. Perjury involves the deliberate misstatement of information while under oath. Lawyers learn that through skillful direct (and cross-) examination of a witness, one can avoid leading a witness into perjury while creating a very different picture from the facts of a case. But, from an ethical viewpoint, there is little difference in the method used if the intent is to deceive (Bakhurst 1992).

People with obsessive-compulsive personality disorder must keep their emotions (particularly anger) as secret as possible, not only from others but also from themselves. This deception is accomplished primarily through the defense mechanism of emotional isolation. Other ego-defense mechanisms used by the obsessive person include rationalization, reaction formation, and projection (see Chapter 2). At times, persons with obsessive-compulsive personality disorder may unconsciously tip their hand and indicate that they have something to hide by using phrases such as "to tell the truth" or "let me be frank with you." This wording suggests that there is, in fact, something hidden (MacKinnon and Michels 1971). Frequently, these people are trying to hide feelings of shame and humiliation or "dirty habits."

Summary

The five persons described in this chapter are all "liars." However, they should not be viewed as immoral or "bad." Patterns in the types of lies told and in the circumstances in which each person is inclined to lie point to the use of lying and self-deception as coping mechanisms. The lies are responses made to deal with the stresses produced by both the external and internal worlds.

Billy Joe, who had an antisocial personality disorder, was truly a professional liar because he used lying as one of his ways to earn a living. Because he did not have a well-developed and internalized sense of right and wrong and because he had very few internal controls, he manipulated the truth and others to obtain instant gratification and to get what he wanted.

Cindy, like Billy Joe, had relatively little guilt about lying. However, she had a histrionic personality disorder and lied for somewhat different purposes: to ingratiate herself to others and to maintain comfort in her interpersonal relationships. She had an intense need for love and approval. Cindy had little respect for the truth, and she exaggerated or rearranged reality for dramatic effect. Both Billy Joe and Cindy were skillful at "reading" other people and being able to determine what other people wanted to hear.

Barbara's lies were a product of her own emotionally distorted inner self. She frequently demonstrated a merging of fantasy and fact. Barbara had a borderline personality disorder, had little control over her impulses, and exercised very little quality control of her statements. At times, wish fulfillment was being expressed; at other times, when she felt hurt or envious, she launched a vicious angry attack.

Marshall lied in an effort to protect his self-esteem. His grandiose aspirations, a feature of narcissistic personality disorder, exceeded his abilities, and he attempted to bridge this gap with prevarication. He was so self-absorbed that he was unable to read his effect on others. He lied not so much to fool others as to deceive himself. As a consequence, his judgment was faulty, and his reality testing was impaired.

The four preceding descriptions of personality disorders (antisocial, histrionic, borderline, and narcissistic) constitute the Cluster B or "dramatic" subtype of personality disorders in DSM-IV. As noted in Chapter 3, some evidence suggests that persons with these personality disorders have neurocognitive deficits that, at least partially, explain some of their symptoms. The deceit of these persons may be facilitated by some difficulty in the temporal organization of memories (the past memory and present fantasy may become fused with current reality), and difficulties in prefrontal-lobe functioning may increase impulsivity and decrease social judgment.

Brooks, who had an obsessive-compulsive personality disorder, deceived himself into thinking that he did not lie. He skillfully provided portions of the truth, while failing to mention essential information, thereby leading others to erroneous conclusions. He used secrecy as a defensive way to maintain his sense of self and to avoid the feeling of being swallowed by others whom he saw as more powerful. Locked in his own secret world, Brooks had a limited capacity to see the "big picture." He functioned well in detail-oriented tasks (such as contracts) but missed out on much in his life.

In conclusion, each of the liars described above processed the day-to-day input and output of information in remarkably different ways. Their lies both reflected and influenced their relationships to life experiences and interpersonal relationships. In the more extreme cases, lying became part of their impaired reality testing.

Chapter 7

Pathological Lying

An awkward, unscientific lie is often as ineffectual as the truth.

—Mark Twain

Many people, particularly those with a strong moralistic bent, regard any lying as pathological. However, as detailed in prior chapters in this book, lying and self-deception are pervasive features of everyday life and human interactions. Furthermore, as I explore in Chapter 13, lying may be beneficial to the individual or may serve the needs of those to whom the lie is directed. In this chapter, *pathological lying* refers to lying that is compulsive or impulsive, occurs on a regular basis, and either does not seem to serve overt material needs of the person or has a self-defeating quality to it. For example, the pathological lie is told even though its ultimate disclosure and negative consequences are inevitable.

The following categories illustrate various forms of pathological lying. They are separated for ease of description and discussion; however, it is obvious that considerable overlap exists among them.

Pseudologia Fantastica

The more extreme forms of pathological lying take the shape of pseudologia fantastica, a matrix of fact and fantasy.

133

■ The Corrupt Judge

Appointed to the bench by Governor George Wallace and reelected by the people of the state of Alabama three times, Judge Jack Montgomery was as colorful as he was controversial (Joynt 1993). He brandished a pistol in his courtroom and used it to threaten both prisoners and lawyers. At one point, he referred to homosexuals as "flame queens" and banned human immunodeficiency virus–infected defendants from his courtroom. He was known for the dramatic war stories he told about himself and for the capriciousness of his sentences. The latter became understandable when the Federal Bureau of Investigation (FBI) instigated a sting operation that culminated in a 1992 warrant to search his home. The FBI discovered thousands of dollars that were allegedly used to bribe him.

Montgomery's subsequent indictment and trial, complete with psychiatric testimony, revealed a great deal about the judge, including the falseness of his stories about himself. He had many tales. He said that he had been the first herpetologist at the Birmingham Zoo, appointed decades ago by the equally colorful Mayor Jimmy Morgan (no such record existed), and that he had been captured and tortured by the Chinese during the Korean War (military records showed that he had never been to Korea). To make the latter story more believable, he refused to eat at Chinese restaurants, citing his past experiences and complaining of nightmares about abuse from the Chinese. These stories were so believable that at one hospital, he received a diagnosis of posttraumatic stress disorder (PTSD). As one psychologist later interpreted his symptoms, he probably did have PTSD, but the cause was his traumatic childhood.

Montgomery was born on Christmas Eve in the rural Louisiana town of Tickfair. His mother was often gone during his childhood. She worked in another town at least 5 days a week, and the future judge lived under the heavy hand of his drunken, abusive father. In later years, he would describe being tied up and beaten with a bullwhip. Although the exact details might be questioned, authorities believed that he had indeed suffered significant physical abuse during his childhood.

During his trial, Judge Montgomery, who had both alcoholism and diabetes, feigned dementia and psychosis. Because he was unable to convince the medical examiners or the presiding judge that he was mentally incompetent, he was convicted. Before his sentencing, he was found dead with a gunshot wound to the head. His death was presumably a suicide, but the weapon was never found.

■ The Glamorous Heiress

Jacqueline, the compulsive liar encountered by Edward Dolnick (1992), was just as flamboyant as Judge Montgomery; however, her case was not as high profile in terms of media coverage. This provocatively dressed petite blond sashayed into Dolnick's life one afternoon and entertained him with accounts of her life for hours. She ultimately confessed that "reality can be so mundane. I try to make it special." Among her numerous tales were stories that she had graduated from Stanford University with a degree in business and a 4.0 grade point average. She also said that she had experienced a dramatic remission from leukemia, the disease that killed her twin sister. Another story was that her boyfriend, who was trying to win her back, had delivered a red Ferrari, tied up with a bow, to her driveway for Christmas. The truth was that she had been a mousy adolescent who nearly flunked out of high school. She experienced sexual abuse and a regretted abortion. To improve her appearance, she had had plastic surgery on her nose and chin and cosmetic work on her teeth. Finally, to boost her self-esteem, she "transformed" (as though she had a fairy godmother) her concerned grandmother into a generous benefactor who provided her with a trust fund and her indifferent boyfriend into a zealous millionaire suitor.

Pseudologia fantastica is a fascinating symptom. The pseudologue spins tales that appear plausible on the surface but do not hang together over time. Fact and fiction are woven together in an interesting matrix until the two are virtually indistinguishable. Unlike a delusional psychotic person, the pseudologue will abandon the story or change it if confronted with contradictory evidence or sufficient disbelief. The stories do have an enduring quality and after repeating them enough times, even the pseudologue begins to believe them (King and Ford 1988).

Brain dysfunction underlies pseudologia fantastica about one-third of the time. For some pseudologues this may take the form of dyslexia or other learning disabilities. Frequently, in those who do have cerebral dysfunction, verbal skills are disproportionately greater than other brain functions, and verbal IQ is higher than performance IQ (King and Ford 1988). It has been suggested that a contributing factor in the production of pseudologia fantastica is that there is a lack of "quality control" for the person's verbal productions (Ford et al. 1988). The more logical and critical portions of the brain (frontal lobes and nondominant hemispheres) fail to monitor verbal output adequately. In the extreme case, this leads to confabulation (see Chapter 3).

Regardless of the importance of cerebral dysfunction in some of these persons, not all pseudologues have evidence of brain damage and not all patients with cerebral dysfunction engage in pseudologia fantastica. Thus, some other explanations for this unique behavior must be considered. Several psychiatrists and psychoanalysts have interpreted pseudologia fantastica from the perspective of unconsciously motivated efforts to preserve or create a sense of self and to defend against overwhelming anxiety.

Helene Deutsch (1921/1982), in a paper that she delivered to the Vienna Psychoanalytic Society more than 70 years ago, viewed pseudologia fantastica as a daydream communicated as reality, often reflecting wishes of an ambitious or erotic nature. Deutsch noted that nearly all people can recall an occasional minor aberration into deception in the course of their truth-loving existence. However, in pseudologia fantastica deception has a pervasive and persistent quality. She further stated that the degree and content of the pseudologia were internally driven rather than produced primarily for the audience. The story of Jacqueline is consistent with Deutsch's formulation, in that Jacqueline created an entire fantasy world, daydreamlike, in order to repress the more painful realities of her past life.

The eminent psychoanalyst and theorist Otto Fenichel (1954) viewed pseudologia fantastica from a different perspective. He proposed that "if it is possible to make someone believe that untrue things are true, then it is also possible that true things, the memory of which threatens me, are untrue" (p. 133). Thus, one purpose of the pseudologia is to avoid thinking about that which is painful or produces anxiety (repression). However, the choice of the subject of the pseudologia may be a disguised form of the painful reality it attempts to hide. Thus, the lie betrays the truth.

The story of Judge Montgomery is an excellent illustration of this hypothesis. He lied repeatedly about abuse associated with being a prisoner of war. In truth he was abused while a "prisoner" of his father during childhood. The painful memories of childhood abuse were displaced into being an abused, but heroic, prisoner of war!

Pseudologia fantastica can also serve a defensive function in helping to maintain a sense of subjective identity and a "viable self." Dithrich (1991) reported on a successful psychoanalysis of an adolescent boy who throughout the course of his analysis repeatedly used pseudologia during the analytic hours. The pseudologia helped the boy distance himself from his depressed, secret-keeping, needy, and intrusive mother. With successful completion of the analysis, the young man was able to look back and say, "I made up all that stuff. It was more interesting than the real me."

Pseudologia fantastica may also be a form of projecting the negative aspects of a person and attributing them to an external object (person). Thus, the fantasies of a person with borderline personality disorder about having been the victim of assault and sexual abuse may be a way of disavowing one's own impulses and attributing them to others (S. Snyder 1986). I discuss false accusations in Chapter 9.

It is often believed that the pseudologue lies effortlessly and with little guilt or emotional arousal. The work of Powell and colleagues (1983), at least with one case, contradicts that perception. A patient, well seasoned in his pseudologia fantastica, demonstrated significant arousal in association with false answers on a polygraph examination. These authors suggested that the pseudologue experiences far more anxiety and guilt than was previously recognized.

Habitual Liars

Most persons who exhibit pathological lying are not as colorful as Judge Montgomery or Jacqueline. Yet, they do inflict considerable pain on those who live or work with them, and they complicate their own lives with their self-defeating behaviors.

■ The Ex-Convict

Freddy, age 24, was brought into the psychiatrist's office by his wife Jackie; she was figuratively holding him by the ear as they came through the door. Jackie immediately announced, "I want you to fix him." The couple had been married fewer than 6 months and, according to Jackie, who was 4 years older than Freddy, she had been the victim of one lie after another. She learned early in their marriage that the honeymoon had been paid for by a loan from Freddy's employer; he had told her that he had saved the money by working overtime. A warrant for parking tickets, which cost $680 to settle, had arrived at the doorstep; Freddy had lied about having paid them. Jackie proceeded to provide a long list of lies around issues such as going to work (he had been fired but did not tell her) and bills (that he said he had paid but had not). She pronounced at one point, "One thing that I know is not a lie is when he tells me that he loves me."

Freddy was a carpet layer, and quite good at it, when he worked. He had just completed parole (2½ years after a brief period in jail for a burglary conviction) when he met Jackie, an installer for the local telephone company. Physically unattractive and with a pugnacious personality, Jackie's matrimonial prospects had been limited. However, Freddy was interested in her and compliant with her various demands, and he promised to "straighten up and fly right," with her help. She also felt sorry for him because of his distress over his prior marriage; his wife had dominated him, frequently belittled him in public, and eventually left him for another man.

Freddy's childhood had been relatively stable. He was likable, quiet, a little shy, and an average student at best. He had not been in disciplinary trouble at school or with the law until he was charged with and convicted for burglary. His previously clean record was the primary reason he had received such a light sentence. Freddy admitted, when seen alone, that his clean record was largely due to luck; he just had not been caught. He had frequently lied to his parents to cover up his use of marijuana and cocaine. He had lied to his first wife and his probation officer about how often he attended Narcotics Anonymous meetings. He lied to his psychotherapist about why he missed scheduled appointments. He said that he really wanted to do better but found himself acting impulsively and then lying to cover up for his behavior.

Freddy's initial response to psychiatric treatment was encouraging. He took his medication (Prozac, prescribed with the goal of reducing impulsivity) and engaged in psychotherapy with the goal of standing up for himself in the marriage rather than lying to avoid confrontation. Interestingly, Jackie called the psychiatrist to complain that he was not as good-natured as he had been and that he had become argumentative. On questioning, she admitted that he was working more regularly and lying less. During a second telephone call, she was more insistent, demanding that Freddy stop taking the medication and that therapy be directed toward making him more compliant with her wishes. She wanted him "fixed," as if there were a diseased part that could be surgically removed. Freddy dropped out of treatment shortly thereafter.

Habitual liars lie for a variety of reasons, some of which were illustrated in the preceding example. There may be an aggressive quality to the lie in an attempt to misguide a rival or take unfair advantage of a situation or another person. In children, lies may serve as a defiant attack on parents, belittling parental values and aspirations. Lies may be efforts to avoid punishment or confrontation. They may also be used to cover up an embarrassing lack of knowledge or merely to entertain oneself or others. Habitual lying may also provide protection from painful feelings caused by a failure to live up to one's own personal standards.

One feature commonly described in compulsive liars is low self-esteem. The lie may be an attempt to feel good about oneself, if only for a short time, much like the effect achieved by abuse of alcohol or other drugs. A repeated lie may bolster self-esteem by displacing blame for one's failure to someone else, or it may create a personal myth of success based on fantasy.

Selling (1942) observed that parental overprotection, sibling rivalry, a dysfunctional family, and mental retardation were among the many causes of pathological lying. The situations described above and in the following chapter illustrate frequently observed psychological aspects to habitual lying. Selling's observations are as accurate today as they were 50 years ago. Persons who are pathological liars repeatedly use deceit as an ego-defense mechanism in an attempt to bolster low self-esteem or to compensate for a lack of more mature ways to cope with everyday problems. This developmental deficit is frequently caused by one or more of the following factors:

- A dysfunctional family of origin
- Childhood physical or sexual trauma
- Neuropsychological abnormalities, including learning disabilities and borderline mental retardation
- Suggestible or accommodating personality features
- Disorders particularly of the sociopathic, borderline, histrionic, and narcissistic types
- Frequent association with substance abuse, either personal or in the family of origin

Lying and Impulse Control Disorders

The impulse control disorders such as pathological gambling, kleptomania, and compulsive shopping are often associated with various forms of deceit.

The Kleptomaniac

Lisa, a 20-year-old unmarried billing clerk, was referred for psychiatric evaluation by the criminal court judge. Lisa, who had previously been placed on probation by the juvenile court, was now being tried as an adult for yet another charge of theft. She had deposited cash payments made to the physician for whom she worked into her own account. Lisa was accompanied to the psychiatric interview by her mother, a well-dressed, upper-middle-class matron who provided additional (and often contradictory) information to that given by Lisa.

Lisa had been charged and convicted of theft twice previously, but those offenses reflected only the times she had been caught and her mother had not been able to successfully intervene. In fact, Lisa had been repeatedly apprehended for shoplifting and had, on several occasions, "borrowed" the credit cards of her friends and her mother, charging thousands of dollars for clothing, jewelry, food, and cosmetics. As a child and young adolescent, Lisa had frequently stolen money from her father's wallet and her mother's purse. Teachers at school had learned that if anything was missing, Lisa's desk or locker was the first place to look. When Lisa was apprehended, her mother would make plausible excuses for Lisa and then pay for whatever loss she had caused. Everyone, including Lisa, agreed that she had no need to steal—her mother was indulgent and provided her with essentially anything she wanted.

Lisa continued, however, to steal and lie repeatedly. Lisa lied about everything—how much money her father earned, how many boyfriends were pursuing her, and how well she was doing at school. When caught stealing, she inevitably had a facile, reasonable excuse for why she had something that did not belong to her. To further complicate her story, Lisa also secretly engaged in bulimia and would, once or twice a week, binge and induce vomiting.

From a psychiatrist's viewpoint, the information about Lisa's family was very revealing. Her father was described as a successful surgeon whose compulsive gambling had led to repeated financial crises that had been kept secret from the children. He was also described by the mother as a "pathological liar" who skillfully covered his absences (to see his bookie) from the hospital and office with plausible excuses. His father (Lisa's paternal grandfather) was an alcoholic, as was Lisa's maternal grandfather.

The overriding dynamic in Lisa's family was the attention provided to her older brother, a professional baseball player. Almost all family activities throughout her childhood had centered around this brother and his athletic accomplishments. Her father may not have been able to take time from his busy medical practice to attend Lisa's piano recitals, but he never missed a Little League or high school baseball game. Lisa's mother doted on the handsome young man, indulged him, and rescued him from his minor misdemeanors.

Lisa was referred for psychological testing that revealed mild dyslexia, in addition to the underlying depression and mixed impulse control disorder (kleptomania, bulimia, and compulsive lying) diagnosed by the psychiatrist. Once again, with the behind-the-scenes interventions of her mother, the judge ordered a brief period of probation and mandated psychiatric treatment. Lisa canceled the first appointment that was scheduled after the end of her probation and never returned for further treatment.

The lying that is frequently observed in persons with impulse control disorders appears to be more pervasive than just the need to cover up behaviors and avoid their consequences. Pathological (or compulsive) lying may itself be an impulse control problem, and thus its association with other difficulties in impulse control may reflect the underlying psychological or brain dysfunction problems common to several syndromes. The impulse control disorders are frequently associated with depression and a personal or family history of substance abuse. McElroy and colleagues (1992) and Stein and colleagues (1993) have suggested that a common neurophysiological abnormality in the impulse control disorders (including the more impulsive personality disorders such as antisocial and borderline personality disorders) is a deficiency in brain serotonin, one of the primary neurotransmitters. Serotonin is known to have inhibitory qualities, and treatment with a medication that increases serotonin at the neural synapse often serves to reduce impulsiveness (McElroy et al. 1992). Clinical research and clinical trials with Prozac or similar medications for treating pathological lying have not yet been reported but might theoretically be helpful.

In addition to neurophysiological substrates to impulsivity, there are also psychological/psychodynamic issues to consider. Goldwater (1994) described impulsive people as deficient in the constructive and preparatory use of fantasy to control their present and their future. They are also only vaguely aware of the past and, thus, live only in the present, for the moment. Goldwater's view of impulsivity is instructive in reference to the lying behaviors of impulsive people. They do not learn from the past and are not aware that other people use the past for reference. Or, in other words, that the truthfulness of the liar's words will be evaluated in terms of past experiences. Furthermore, the impulsive liar fails to take into account the various effects (including negative effects on the liar himself or herself) that a lie may produce. As a result, the impulsive person lies to gratify current feelings and thoughts without regard to either the past or the future.

Lying and Substance Abuse

All physicians are acutely aware of the high frequency of lying in patients with substance abuse.

■ The Sales Manager

"Can do! The shipment will be there next Thursday." Dan glibly promised the purchasing agent of another company that his firm would make delivery of the overdue computer programs. He then hung up the telephone and put his head on the desk. "Oh, my God, I've done it again." He looked around the office piled high with requisition requests and other bits and pieces of unfiled correspondence. He was weeks behind in his work, and the telephone calls and complaints kept coming. Eager to please and unable to say no, he continued to make promises far beyond his ability to keep.

Dan spent the remainder of the afternoon fielding complaints from customers and providing glib outward charm. His apparent sincerity convinced most of these people that he was genuinely trying to help and would meet their needs. He intended to work late to reduce his backlog but at 5 o'clock decided that he needed a good night's sleep in order to get a jump the next day on his problems. On the way home, he stopped at his favorite bar, "to relax and have a drink." Three hours and six drinks later he arrived home to a chronically disappointed wife, ate a warmed-over dinner, and fell into bed. Her sexual advances were once again rejected with, "Honey, I'm just too tired and stressed out from work." He awoke the next morning to a day that proceeded and ended much as had the previous days.

Dan's continued employment as sales manager was a frequent matter of discussion by his superior, a corporate vice president. He liked Dan, as did almost everyone, but the enthusiasm with which he had been hired had faded. Somehow the job just was not getting done. The excuses always made sense, but there were so many of them. Sales were also falling below predictions. Despite his complaints of overwork, he often came in late and left early. Moreover, there was a growing discomfort that some of his stories were contradictory or inconsistent. For example, at one time, he had said that he was in Vietnam during 1972. At another time, he said that he was playing football that year at a well-known southern university. Word had also come in that indicated the performance at his previous place of employment, which he had described as stellar, was actually unsatisfactory.

Dan was the younger of two children born to the family of a small-town hardware store owner. He was always in the shadow of an older, attractive, bright sister whom he adored because she provided much of his maternal care. His mother was emotionally unavailable, both because of her work as a real estate agent and because she was a closet alcoholic. To please his father, Dan played football in high school, well enough to be All-State second string. His friendly, cheerful manner was recognized in the high school yearbook label of "most popular boy" in the senior class.

Unfortunately, Dan's athletic ambitions and academic goals at college were not sufficient to overcome the temptations of fraternity life and the almost endless beer parties. He left college on academic probation after only two semesters and enlisted in the United States Army Reserve. His service record was marked by a lackluster performance as a supply clerk and disciplinary action for alcohol abuse. He returned to a small state college, from which he received a degree in marketing. He met his wife, Betty, while in college, and although she had some concerns about his drinking, she assumed that it was "just a phase." Indeed, early in their marriage, Dan's drinking was fairly well controlled, but as the years progressed and the responsibilities of family and home ownership increased, so did his drinking. Neither of the couple would have called him an "alcoholic"; he had never been arrested for driving under the influence, had never had delirium tremens, and had never missed a day at work. But Dan was, in fact, an alcoholic—one of countless thousands of middle- or upper-middle-class persons who do not fit the stereotype and whose social skills and type of work disguise their abuse of alcohol.

Dan hid the knowledge of his alcoholism from himself, and Betty used rationalization and her own self-deception to deny it. Like many families with an alcoholic member, they invested considerable energy in maintaining the facade of normality. Dan finally came to psychiatric attention when, after being fired from his job, he became suicidally depressed. He still continued to deny his alcoholism, however.

Most, if not all, people who abuse alcohol or other drugs engage in considerable deceit—both of themselves and others. Lying is such a prominent feature of alcoholism that addressing it is an important part of the Alcoholics Anonymous program (Alcoholics Anonymous World Services 1976). Members are urged to be truthful not only about present activities but also about prior deceptions.

In their study of recovery from alcoholism, Strom and Barone (1993) found that self-deception typifies the active abuser. Active alcoholic persons maintain high self-esteem and the belief that they can control their drinking. In contrast, those in late recovery (i.e., sober for more than 1 year) feel good about themselves but demonstrate significantly less self-deception. It seems probable that an important part of addiction recovery is learning how to be more honest with oneself and with others.

The alcoholic individual is not the only person to engage in self-deception and lying. Such deceit pervades the entire family, and both the addict and family members begin to believe their own lies (Krestan and Bepko 1993). The lifestyle of the alcoholic person is one of lying, secrecy, and ultimately silence. The entire family is drawn into this net, and all family relationships become dominated by lying and secrecy. In the absence of honest exchange of emotional feelings, intimacy is lost. Such conditions may have long-term effects on children who were reared in alcoholic homes.

That people who are addicted to drugs deceive physicians in their drug-seeking behavior is both well known and problematic (Pancratz et al. 1989). Patients may claim to have lost their medication or misunderstood prescription directions so that they can obtain early prescription refills. These patients may see many physicians concurrently in order to obtain more medications for use or for sale. Pancratz and colleagues related the story of one postoperative patient who claimed he was due for more surgery. He stated that he lived in another city and needed hydromorphine to "tide him over." Careful investigation disclosed that he had obtained thousands of opiate tablets in this manner.

A British physician (McKeganey 1988) stated that physicians are reluctant to become involved with opiate users because of their persistent lying. This deceit undermines any potential benefit from the doctor-patient relationship. McKeganey was less pessimistic about alcoholic patients, whom he regarded as deceitful about their drinking behavior but honest enough for the doctor to gain some grasp of their situation.

Denial (self-deception) remains a key part of the addictive process. Addicted people lie to themselves and to others in an effort to avoid exposure, shame, and humiliation; they also lie to others (including physicians) to obtain the desired substance. Ultimately, the deceit involves the entire family and social system, which causes significant secondary effects on all.

Summary

Pathological lying covers a wide spectrum of severity, from habitual lying in certain circumstances to pervasive pseudologia fantastica. Lying is a frequently found clinical feature associated with the impulse control disorders (e.g., kleptomania, gambling, and compulsive shopping) and with substance abuse.

The childhood histories of persons with pathological lying often include physical or sexual abuse, dysfunctional families, impulsive behavior, low self-esteem, and dyslexia or other forms of cerebral dysfunction. The etiological role of these factors is unclear, but—separately or in combination—genetic predisposition, cerebral dysfunction, and the lack of a secure childhood may facilitate the emergence of chronic lying as a maladaptive coping mechanism.

Chapter 8

Living a Lie: Impostors, Con Artists, and Persons With Munchausen Syndrome

I am a superior sort of liar. I don't tell any truth at all.

—Ferdinand Demara

Impostors represent the extreme end of the continuum of pathological liars. They continuously live a lie, to the point of assuming new names and identities for each role they play. For some there is a con-artist quality to their posturing; for others, the only identifiable goal of the imposture is the thrill of pulling it off. Patients with Munchausen syndrome deceive doctors and pose as medical patients; they have many similarities to impostors.

In this chapter, I recount the stories of several impostors, con artists, and Munchausen patients and interpret their behavior from a psychological perspective.

Impostors

The medical literature contains several detailed life stories of impostors who have been psychiatrically studied (Deutsch 1955; DuPont 1970; Finkelstein 1974; Wijsenbeek and Nitzan 1968). The following stories have been gleaned from the many stories about impostors that have been published in the lay press.

■ The Great Impostor

The most famous impostor of this century, perhaps in history, was Ferdinand Waldo Demara (1922–1982). Demara's exploits became nationally known in 1952 after a major article in *Life* magazine (McCarthy 1952). He had recently been revealed as posing as a physician and medical officer in the Royal Canadian Navy. His exposure had occurred, not because of medical incompetence, but because of his widely publicized successes in the surgical treatment of severely wounded Koreans. The operations were performed aboard the Canadian naval destroyer *Cayuga*, to which Demara was assigned; the surgery included procedures such as the removal of a bullet lodged within half an inch of the heart and a pneumectomy (removal of a lung). Despite the widespread notoriety associated with this imposture, Demara was discharged from the Royal Canadian Navy (rather than facing court-martial) with a check for back pay due to him. He was not so lucky with some other prior endeavors and twice served time in correctional facilities, once for posing as a teacher and once for deserting the United States Army. While absent without leave from the army, he enlisted in the United States Navy and then deserted from the navy—he was a simultaneous deserter from both the army and navy! His experiences in the armed services later served him well in impersonating a naval physician.

An investigation of Demara's background led to the discovery that at various times he had impersonated a Ph.D. in psychology, a college dean, a schoolteacher, and an assistant warden of a Texas prison. Amazingly, according to the best information, he competently completed his responsibilities in each of these roles. When discovered, or bored, he would return home to his parents in Lawrence, Massachusetts. He appeared to maintain a satisfactory relationship with them, and the degree of their knowledge of his activities was not established.

Publicity created by the *Life* article led to the publication of Demara's biography by Robert Crichton (1959a), a best-seller that was later made into the 1960 movie, *The Great Impostor*, with Tony Curtis in the title role. Crichton (1959b) later wrote another book about his travels, interactions, and frustrations in dealing with Demara to gather data for the biography.

Demara's childhood history, as can best be determined, was initially one of warmth, love, and riches. He was large in size, demanded things his way, went into rages when frustrated, and often felt unaccepted by other boys. He was an acolyte in the Roman Catholic church and was considered a candidate for the priesthood. When Demara was 11 years old, his father lost everything he owned, which placed the family in poverty. When he was 15, his sister Elaine died of a head injury. A depression settled over the house, and less than a month later Demara ran away from home to join a Trappist monastery.

Following the fame brought by his biography and the movie, Demara again returned to a life of imposture for several years before becoming a hospital chaplain under his own name. He died of heart failure in 1982 at age 60 (Sifakis 1993).

Demara was clearly a brilliant man who could have succeeded at almost anything he wished. Why did he instead choose to be an impostor in a variety of roles? The reasons are speculative—Demara himself, when asked, "Why?," responded with "Because I am a rotten man." He then added, "It's rascality, pure rascality." Obviously it was not that simple, and during his various impostures, he often behaved in an altruistic manner.

■ The Fighter Pilot

"As an old fighter pilot, I'll bomb that guy out of the saddle." An arrogant, brash political mover who had "broken kneecaps all over town," Duke Tully's language was full of allusions to his distinguished military career. His home was full of plaques, medals, and pictures celebrating his wartime experiences in Korea and Vietnam. At social functions, he wore the uniform of a United States Air Force lieutenant colonel, decorated with the Purple Heart, the Air Medal with four oak leaf clusters, and the Distinguished Flying Cross. "He was like an officer in life," said one friend about Tully, whose political power came from his management of two large southwestern newspapers. Almost inevitably, Tully crossed one political rival too many, one who checked his credentials and exposed him. In truth, Tully had never been in the military (Alter and Collier 1986).

Tully's impersonation began around age 20, when he joined the Civil Air Patrol and started wearing a uniform. "I started to tell a fib and one fib led to another . . . I helped it grow. Once it got going, it just picked up steam, and I fed it." Tully changed jobs several times and each time "promoted" himself in his employment applications, from second lieutenant to major to lieutenant colonel. With the moves and promotions, Tully embellished the war stories with multiple missions, an airplane crash, and decorations. Both his first wife (who died young) and his second wife, as well as his children, had believed the stories, and he had been publicly honored by several military organizations. One friend who attempted to analyze Tully's behavior commented that Tully had lost several family members (including his first wife) to war or illness and had reacted by trying to shore himself up against more tragedy by making himself a strong person. Another acquaintance noted Tully's need for approval, attention, and adulation. He needed to be the center of attention.

The paradox of this story is that Tully's actual accomplishments were considerable. He was literate, well-read, and had risen from a $38-a-week classified advertising sales position to publisher of two of Arizona's largest newspapers. His newspapers, influenced by his conservative editorial positions, formed a powerful political base, and he was also a major force in expanding the arts in Phoenix. Why should such an obviously talented man need to perpetuate a charade that would bring such embarrassment on disclosure? Tully himself provided relatively little information. However, it is apparently significant that an older brother, whom Tully had idolized, was a fighter pilot killed in World War II.

■ The Munchausen Expert

When Dr. Ganesh Patel (pseudonym) arrived in Australia, he was warmly welcomed into the group of psychiatric experts who worked with medical and surgical patients. His credentials looked excellent, and he said that his father and grandfather were major political figures in his native India. Dr. Patel had come from the United States, where he reported that he had run a group for Munchausen patients (see below). Dr. Patel began a research project that, because of irregularities, came under close scrutiny and an official investigation. His "research" was found to contain fabricated data, as did his curriculum vitae. His resignation was accepted; Dr. Patel was not finished, however. He published a letter (patently false) in a leading British medical journal stating that the investigation had cleared him. A more recent article in a Canadian newspaper stated that the physician, now in Canada, had been nominated for a Nobel Prize. This information, apparently leaked by Dr. Patel, also proved to be a fabrication. The ironic part of Dr. Patel's story was that he (a master prevaricator) had styled himself as an expert in treating deceitful patients.

The three impostors described above were obviously of highly superior intellect. They demonstrated that they had a capacity for achievement and could have been recognized for their own abilities and accomplishments, under their own names. Why did they choose to assume roles in which they ultimately betrayed themselves? Both laypersons and psychological experts have sought answers to these questions about impostors in general. The best hypotheses come from some distinguished psychoanalysts who, through their personal clinical work and scholarship, have carefully studied the phenomenon of imposture.

Greenacre (1958a) noted the paucity of female impostors and speculated that the psychodynamics of women are different and may lead to other conditions related to imposture such as malingering. Greenacre related the history (of uncertain accuracy) of a woman in the ninth century who impostured a priest and ultimately became the pope. Some historical accounts record her as "Pope Joan." Irrespective of whether imposture occurs in women—and it apparently does, as illustrated by the fact that women do exhibit the Munchausen syndrome (see below)—there are no psychoanalytic descriptions of women impostors per se. Therefore, the following descriptions of psychological motivations relate to men.

A classic paper by Karl Abraham (1935), one of the early psychoanalysts, reported a man whom Abraham had first seen in the course of his duties as a military physician. At that time, the man was identified as a swindler who had repeatedly impersonated officers and obtained money under false pretenses. Abraham had the opportunity to see the man 5 years later and found him to be a changed man. In the interim, the swindler had married an older widow whom he called "little mother." She had recognized his talent and helped him rise to a responsible position in the family business; he took the place of her dead husband. Abraham interpreted these fortuitous circumstances as allowing the man to live out his oedipal wishes in an acceptable way, with less guilt because the husband was dead, and the woman had taken the initiative. Oedipal issues (as will be seen in the following discussion), feelings of impotence (castration fears), and an insecure sexual identity have been common psychoanalytic interpretations of the unconscious determinants of imposture.

Several characteristics of the childhood and developmental experiences of impostors have been observed. For example, an unusually close relationship with an overinvolved, intrusive mother has been described (Deutsch 1955; DuPont 1970; Finkelstein 1974). At times, both parents have been described as doting and providing an audience for the child to show off (Crichton 1959a; Finkelstein 1974). As a child, the future impostor often seems to be precocious and aware of his or her effect on others. Both the family and the child have high expectations for achievement and future success. The father of the future impostor has frequently been described as a man whose wealth and power would be impressive to a boy, influencing the expectations and aspirations of the son.

This particular constellation (an overinvolved mother and powerful father) intensifies infantile narcissism and provides fertile ground for significant oedipal conflict. The boy fears retaliation from the father for usurping the attentions of the mother. In most situations, this conflict is resolved when the boy develops a healthy identification with the father. However, if there are adverse circumstances in the family's life, successful resolution of the oedipal conflict might not occur. The father might be absent or disinterested, or he might be rendered powerless through illness or bankruptcy (Crichton 1959a; Deutsch 1955; DuPont 1970). This particular scenario is apparent in the description of Demara (Crichton 1959a), whose family experienced severe financial reverses. The failure of the father or his absence results in devaluation and an incomplete masculine identification, with subsequent failure to master the developmental steps needed for ego maturation. One other circumstance, noted by Greenacre (1958a), in historically significant impostors is that many were physically or sexually impaired.

Based on the above factors that seem to influence the development of imposture, Finkelstein (1974) has interpreted imposture as the individual's need to appear in grandiose roles in an attempt to overcome narcissistic problems of low self-esteem. Deutsch (1955) also emphasized the role of imposture as an attempt to eliminate the friction between the impostor's pathologically exaggerated ego ideal and a "devaluated inferior guilt-laden part of his ego" (p. 503). The imposture is necessary because the individual's ego is devalued when expressed in his own name. In other words, the impostures serve the purpose of transiently creating the powerful masculine image to which the impostor aspires. Through the imposture, the man unconsciously usurps the role of the father, but the resulting guilt often results in his betrayal of this assumed role.

The psychoanalytic view presented above emphasizes the oedipal conflict, with imposture representing an acting-out behavior in an effort to resolve internal tension. Other perspectives place less emphasis on oedipal issues. For example, imposture may be an attempt to define oneself and to create an identity and a sense of self. Some impostors describe a feeling of emptiness when they are themselves and a feeling of energy and vitality when successfully playing a role. This may be particularly important for those individuals who have a perception of (or perhaps a genuine physical disability leading to) genital inadequacy (Conrad 1975). Dr. Roy Grinker, Jr., (1961) believed that imposture might be an attempt to master a past failure, thus restoring a sense of competence. The individual with low self-esteem, who envies those perceived as more competent, may achieve a feeling of superiority through successfully fooling others by devaluing those who have been taken in. Through successfully duping others, the one who is weak becomes strong and superior.

Living a lie may also serve to deny painful reality. As noted in Chapter 7, Fenichel (1954) proposed that if one can make someone else believe something that is not true, then perhaps something that has occurred in the past may not be true. This process is best illustrated by Demara's own words:"I am a superior sort of liar. I don't tell any truth at all, so then my story has unity of parts, a structural integrity, and this sounds more like the truth than the truth itself" (qtd. in Crichton 1968, p. 92). In this regard, the role of imposture as a defense against depression must also be considered (C. N. Lewis 1990). The personal histories of many impostors point to a significant loss just before the onset of the imposture. The imposture may serve to deny the loss and, through the enormous psychic energy required for the successful imposture, may defend the impostor from painful feelings. In fact, much as with mania, impostors describe a feeling of exhilaration as they successfully become a new person. Crichton (1959b) described Demara as behaving with an energized, almost manic manner; yet one of Demara's closest friends, a physician, called him "the most miserable, unhappy man I have known" (Garvey 1985, p. 21).

Greenacre (1958b) compared the impostor to the artist; in a certain sense, imposture can be seen as an artistic performance. Although there is certainly no single explanation for creativity, it does appear that the creative work of some artists (e.g., Edvard Munch, Rene Magritte) has been motivated by the need to deny and overcome intense feelings of loss and emptiness (Viederman 1987; Warick and Warick 1984). To quote Greenacre (1958b, p. 540), "In both creative artist on the brink of a new surge of creativity and the impostor between periods of imposture, there is a sense of ego hunger and a need for completion—in the one, of the artistic self; in the other, of a satisfying identity in the world."

Impostors are certainly interesting to many people. Newspapers and popular magazines periodically report the disclosure of a new impostor who has been playing a dramatic or important role. Part of our interest in imposture stems from universal questions and feelings about personal identity that each of us has. Deutsch (1955) commented on the blurring of the boundaries between pathology and normalcy. She observed that "the world is crowded with 'as-if' personalities, and even more so with impostors and pretenders. Ever since I became interested in the impostor, he pursues me everywhere. I find him among my friends and acquaintances, as well as in myself" (p. 503).

Every child has played a variety of make-believe roles and dress-up games. In addition, all adults have probably questioned their public personae in terms of their private personal identity. Many successful people feel that they are frauds or impostors and not really as capable and competent as others may think. This constellation of thoughts and feelings has become known as the *impostor syndrome*. It was described by Conrad (1975) as a neurotic response to an underlying feeling of inadequacy. He observed that these people are afraid to become close to others for fear that their weaknesses will be disclosed.

The impostor phenomenon was popularized by Clance and Imes (1978; Clance 1985) as characteristic of certain high-achieving women who perceive themselves as frauds. Subsequently, the syndrome has been shown to include both sexes and to have some relation to types of self-defeating behaviors (Kets de Vries 1990). Persons with the impostor syndrome feel that they have fooled everybody and are not as competent or intelligent as others think they are. They feel like frauds or impostors, attributing their success to luck, physical attractiveness, likability, or compensatory hard work. They may have been more successful than their parents and moved into a higher-status social class, and this discrepancy between their origins and their new roles may increase their feelings of being impostors.

Confidence Artists

The following description of a self-proclaimed "con man" was obtained from his autobiography, which was produced with the assistance of a professional writer (Abagnale 1980).

■ The Master Con Artist

When last heard from, Frank Abagnale, Jr., impostor and master con man, was "honestly" the head of a firm that specialized in teaching employees of businesses and banks how to identify and avoid white-collar crime. Abagnale's career as a confidence man began at age 14, when he conned his father out of thousands of dollars with a credit card scheme. He subsequently impersonated a Pan American pilot and repeatedly flew for free on international flights. At one point, he was offered the opportunity (as a courtesy) to take the controls of an overseas airliner. Even though he had never had a flying lesson in his life, he briefly sat in the pilot's seat and bluffed his way through a potentially disastrous situation. As a result of his numerous scams, which allowed him to lead a luxurious lifestyle, he was ultimately apprehended and served time in French, Swedish, and American prisons.

In his autobiography, Abagnale provides little information about his childhood and adolescence, other than that his parents had a poor relationship and separated when he was 12 years old. His father often asked him to play the role of mediator between the parents. Abagnale describes his father as a successful businessman who drank constantly and was indulgent to the adolescent Abagnale. The father had major financial reverses during Abagnale's teenage years.

Note that Abagnale's entire autobiography, from the title (*Catch Me If You Can*) to the last sentence, reeks of self-satisfied pleasure at his cleverness and skill at putting something over on others (his victims). This characteristic illustrates Ekman's (1992) description of *duping delight*. To quote Abagnale, "I'm still a con artist. I'm just putting down a positive con these days, as opposed to the negative con I used in the past. I have simply redirected the talents I've always possessed" (p. 253).

■ The Con Lady

None of the parishioners of St. Stephen's had an inkling that the genteel cultured woman they had just elected church treasurer would soon defraud the church of $20,000. They certainly did not know that this charming, attractive woman had already served 2½ years in the state women's prison for embezzling $1.2 million from the bond brokerage firm where she had been employed as an account executive.

Sheri had all the attributes of a southern lady. She asked about others' grandchildren, baked cakes for the church bazaar, dressed demurely with only a single string of small pearls for jewelry, and lived in the elite part of the city among the "old," established families. She was, however, an "ex-con," in more than one way.

Sheri used her simple, winning ways, combined with complete self-confidence, to fool those around her. It was not clever bookkeeping techniques that enabled her to divert substantial amounts of money into her personal banking accounts but rather a lack of suspicion. She was caught each time by carelessness that, in retrospect, seemed to be unconsciously motivated self-defeating behavior.

Sheri recalled her childhood as relatively pleasant until age 5 years, when her father had abandoned the family. Her mother then began to have violent outbursts, punctuated with accusations that the father had left because he couldn't stand living with the children. Following these abusive episodes, the mother would pretend that they had not occurred. Sheri started to lie to avoid her mother's beatings, and soon deceit became a way of life for her. She changed the grades on her report card, wrote excuses forging her mother's signature for school absences, and began to shoplift. Concurrently, and seemingly incongruent with the above behaviors, Sheri's social skills and personal attractiveness continued to develop and she effectively hid her "dark side" from boyfriends. She was married at age 18 to a solid, but uninteresting, young man who was unaware of her family's secrets.

Sheri's embezzlements began 3 years later. They were the product of both a need for more money and of her boredom with the marriage. When she was apprehended, her husband initially disbelieved the claims against her, but he quietly sought a divorce following her conviction and imprisonment. After release from prison, Sheri created a new personal history to hide information about her prior life from the men with whom she had a series of relationships. Interestingly, she would react with rage if she caught a suitor lying to her.

From a psychodynamic perspective, Sheri—a product of a markedly dysfunctional family—learned in childhood how to compartmentalize her life. She effectively presented herself to the world as an attractive, cultured, and competent woman, but inwardly she felt damaged and unlovable. Her skill at lying and fraud provided transient feelings of mastery and power, but even when she was being ostensibly successful, her devalued sense of self would undermine her success and lead to failure.

Relatively little is known about the psychological makeup of confidence men or women, despite the interest they create in the lay press and media. A large number of books have been published about confidence men (Hyman 1989), but these books—including the classic *The American Confidence Man* (Maurer 1974)—focus on details of various scams and colorful descriptions of these under-world people, rather than on the psychological factors that motivate behavior.

Among the meager empirical data available is the work by S. B. G. Eysenck and colleagues (1977), who found that men convicted of confidence crimes (fraud) differed significantly from other criminals as evaluated by the Eysenck Personality Questionnaire. The former tended to have low psychoticism scale scores, high extroversion scores, and low neuroticism scores. These findings are exactly the opposite of the scores of those criminals convicted of common theft.

Con artists are known as the aristocrats of the criminal world. They tend to have high intelligence; are suave, slick, and capable; and tend to prosper through their superb knowledge of human nature. "Relatively few good con men are ever brought to trial; of those who are tried, few are convicted; of those who are convicted, even fewer serve out their full sentence" (Maurer 1974, p. 3).

The few discussions of con artists in the psychoanalytic literature are often linked with impostors, although there is little in the way of firm data to establish this connection. This connection seems intuitively reasonable because the con artist is pretending to be something that he or she is not. Inferences about developmental and psychodynamic issues have often been drawn from analysis of novels such as Thomas Mann's *Confessions of Felix Krull, Confidence Man* and Herman Melville's *The Confidence-Man* (Gray 1975; Kets de Vries 1990). Gray's interpretation of the psychological workings of the confidence man is especially innovative and provocative. He describes the con artist as like the psychotherapist, individualizing the approach and tailoring his or her words to the particular foibles and illusions of the subject. Gray goes on to say that good con artists, like hypnotists, must con themselves into believing—even temporarily—the scheme they are proposing. This assists in building a relationship of illusionary intimacy. Gray viewed the con artist as being motivated by greed; having a voracious appetite; and seeking to possess another person's money, allegiance, or sense of self. The con artist craves to possess people through the confidential relationship, and this characteristic may lead some of these individuals into politics or evangelical preaching.

The confidence game appears to be a dynamic relationship built on the needs of the "mark" as well as those of the exploiter. The con artist has an almost uncanny ability to discover the victim's vulnerable areas and to "pitch the con" to those areas. Yet, despite their successful manipulation of others, they often engage in self-defeating behavior that ultimately trips them up.

Hankiss (1980) outlined techniques to run a con; she described placing the "bait" and ways to make it appear authentic. These tactics include providing irrelevant or extraneous information, some of which the mark will know to be true and some of which will make the story sound more convincing. The con artist convinces the victim of the former's version of reality by playing on the latter's stereotyped expectations of reality and on psychodynamic or sociodynamic factors. For example, people are reluctant to challenge another person's honesty openly. The skillful con artist learns to disarm suspicions by bringing them up first, anticipating the victim's own doubts. Similarly, the con artist will make efforts to establish a connection with the mark—for example, something shared in the past, a common friend or relative, or a similar religious persuasion. With the usual expectation that most people are trustworthy, this common link helps to dispel any doubts. Thus, the con artist enters the person's life and takes something away.

Medical Impostors

The impostors described above primarily assumed roles in which they were important people (e.g., physicians, military officers) who deserved respect and admiration. The person who simulates a disease is also an impostor but one who is assuming the role of patient. In American society, the sick role relieves people of their usual responsibilities and, to a large extent, demands that other persons give care.

Munchausen Syndrome

Munchausen syndrome was originally described in a delightfully whimsical article by Richard Asher (1951), a British physician. The syndrome has three major features: the dramatic simulation of disease, pseudologia fantastica, and peregrination (wandering from hospital to hospital). The Munchausen patient often uses a variety of aliases. One of these "patients" has been documented to have been admitted to hospitals more than 400 times, amassing enormous medical care costs (von Maur et al. 1973). The following case histories highlight many of the characteristics of these patients.

■ The Frequent Flyer

A large commercial airliner rolled up to the gate area of the small midwestern airport, and an ambulance, lights flashing, drove out on the tarmac to meet it. The ground crew pushed the stairway up to the door and the paramedics, carrying a stretcher, rushed up and entered the plane. A few moments later, they emerged carrying a thin, blond young man writhing in pain and strapped to the stretcher. They placed him in the ambulance and sped away. Meanwhile, the airline returned to the end of the runway to take off. Its coast-to-coast flight had been interrupted by a medical emergency; or was it an emergency?

Stevie had struck again! Stevie has flown all over North America and has been hospitalized in Fairbanks, Alaska; Honolulu, Hawaii; and Miami, Florida—to mention only a few of his many hospital stays. He has a remarkable ability to mimic renal colic (a kidney stone in the ureter causing excruciating pain). He has twice been the cause of airliners making unscheduled emergency stops in order for him to be taken to a hospital. However, renal colic is only one example from his repertoire of simulated diseases. He can feign symptoms that indicate the need for an emergency surgical procedure with such conviction that his belly looks like a "road map" from the multitude of surgical scars. He has mastered the simulation of acute intermittent porphyria, Mediterranean fever, and regional ileitis.

After his ruse was discovered during one hospitalization, Stevie allowed himself to be transferred to a psychiatric unit. His mother was contacted, and the following story emerged from information collected from the two of them (neither was regarded as a very reliable historian).

Stevie was the only child born to a career-oriented professional woman and a medically disabled father. The mother traveled extensively, so most of Stevie's childcare needs were met by his kind and lenient father. Stevie had difficulties in early childhood with neuropathic traits that included nail biting, habitual lying, and poor relationships with other children. At age 8, he was placed in a residential facility for disturbed children. While he was there, his father died; after Stevie returned home for the funeral, he was placed in a series of foster homes. He received infrequent visits from his mother, who periodically sent him expensive gifts ("to buy me off").

He eventually graduated from high school, but he flunked out of college after less than 2 years. He then sought out his mother who was living in a different state, moved in, and established a love-hate relationship with her. His Munchausen behavior would characteristically be triggered by her departure on a business trip. He reported that he would feel rejected and enormously anxious and would then simulate an illness in order to gain admission to a local hospital.

Stevie often used an alias and made up various stories about himself, such as being a junior executive. When he had exhausted the available local hospitals (he had become too well known), he began taking airplane trips to different North American cities and fraudulently gaining admission to hospitals in cities where he was unknown. During his admission to the psychiatric unit, Stevie proved to be a superb actor. He would assume different roles and play the parts, dressed in the appropriate wardrobe, in a very convincing manner. Among these roles were the junior executive, complete with a three-piece suit and wing-tip shoes; the tennis club pro, with tennis whites and a racket; and "Joe College," nonchalantly sloppy in a famous midwestern university sweat shirt.

Psychological testing revealed superior intelligence, creativity, and no cerebral dysfunction in an immature, passive, ineffectual personality. There was no evidence of psychosis or major depression. Efforts to establish a close relationship and engage him in psychotherapy were futile. Despite his superficial likability, there was a fearful, guarded inner core that regarded the world as a hostile, dangerous place. He eventually bolted from treatment, presumably to seek a medical admission at another hospital.

■ The Bereaved Daughter

A psychiatry resident physician, the seasoned veteran of hundreds of inner-city emergency room consultations, found himself trying to wipe tears from his eyes inconspicuously as he listened to the tragic story. "They were so good. I miss them so much." The slightly disheveled middle-aged woman cried profusely as she told of the deaths of her parents in a recent automobile accident. She had been following them home in her own car late one night, when suddenly another car had veered across the double line and crashed head-on into the car of her parents. She had reached the accident scene only to see the mangled bodies and hear their agonal moans.

The accident had occurred weeks ago, but Rose could not get it off her mind, and the images were as vivid as if it had happened yesterday. Furthermore, she couldn't sleep well because of recurring nightmares. The sizable inheritance she had received from her parents was "meaningless," and she had lost 30 pounds. Rose reported that she was actively considering suicide but had decided, late that night, to seek help in the emergency room, and the psychiatry resident on call had been summoned to further evaluate her.

Rose was immediately admitted to the psychiatry ward, and she provided further information of a heart-rending nature. An intruder had entered her home the previous week, had assaulted her, and started to rape her before being frightened off by sounds of the neighbor returning home. She had also lost a child to leukemia in the past. Everyone's heart went out to this woman who seemed to have no end to misfortune.

According to the history provided by Rose, she was an only child born to a Polish couple who had emigrated to the United States following World War II when she was a small child. They had struggled to learn English, and Rose had been teased by schoolmates because of her accent. However, by virtue of their hard work, her parents had established a thriving electrical supply wholesale company. After high school graduation, Rose attended college for a brief time before marrying a well-to-do southern gentleman who changed after their marriage. He became an alcoholic and philanderer. Following the death of their only child, she decided to return to her parents' home, where she had continued to live for a number of years.

As time progressed during Rose's hospitalization, it became increasingly apparent that many aspects of her story were false. The ward staff were also concerned that she was rarely visited by friends, and those who did visit left too quickly to be questioned. The ward psychiatrists became suspicious about the story of the parental deaths and asked the local newspaper to check their files. No report of a fatal accident or listing in the obituaries was found that could confirm Rose's story. Rose was gently confronted with this information and, with information from some relatives, her tale gradually unraveled.

The more accurate history was that Rose was one of several children born to a southern country family. Her childhood was marked by abuse, both physical and sexual, by an alcoholic father and neglect by a tired, disinterested mother. Rose was a bright and verbal child who graduated from high school and was married several times. Her only child, a daughter, would have nothing to do with her. Rose's finances were always marginal; she had been arrested several times for prostitution and had been incarcerated in the state's prison for women for prescription fraud.

Of considerable interest to Rose's psychiatric physicians was the discovery that she had been previously admitted to the same large teaching hospital on multiple occasions, using different names, for physical complaints that were never proven to have an organic cause. She had also been admitted to other local hospitals, using different names, at various times. The hospital admission described above, and many preceding it, had been precipitated by a breakup with her live-in male companion.

Patients with Munchausen syndrome and its less extreme companion, simple factitious disorder (see section, "Simple Factitious Disorder," below), are fascinating in that, superficially, their behavior makes so little sense. Who would want to be sick and in a hospital? Furthermore, who would deliberately submit to obviously unneeded surgical procedures when no financial or other gain is apparent? Various authors have looked for common threads in the life circumstances and psychological constitutions of Munchausen patients in an effort to understand this bizarre behavior.

More than 20 years ago, I summarized the phenomenological data then available about both childhood and adult characteristics of Munchausen syndrome (Ford 1973). Hundreds, perhaps thousands, of published case reports since then have generally confirmed those earlier observations. The childhood experiences of the Munchausen patient frequently included a rejecting or sadistic parent, an association with death or chronic illness in the childhood home, bizarre or neurotic childhood behavior, and an episode of institutionalization or hospitalization. Of note, Munchausen patients frequently regarded their childhood hospitalization as a positive experience because it rescued the child from an unhappy home situation, at least temporarily.

The adult life experiences and characteristics of Munchausen patients included the presence of severe personality disorders (especially of the borderline and antisocial types), poor work histories, work in health-related jobs when working, suicide attempts, and psychiatric hospitalization. The experience of loss or rejection as precipitating Munchausen behavior has also been noted on numerous occasions.

A number of etiologies for Munchausen syndrome have been proposed (M. D. Feldman and Ford 1994; Ford 1973, 1982, 1983; Spivak et al. 1994). For many patients, the behavior of Munchausen syndrome may be meeting many needs at the same time. The following description has been developed from the work of many authors but should not be regarded as exhaustive of various potential etiologies.

- *Food and shelter:* Among the earliest explanations for Munchausen behavior was that patients were essentially homeless people looking for a place to stay. Basic needs were met in return for playing the sick role. In the 1990s, however, this does not seem to be a prominent reason for seeking hospitalization.
- *Drug-seeking behavior:* It has been observed that many Munchausen patients simulate illnesses or symptoms that require opiates. It has been proposed that the Munchausen behavior is an elaborate drug-seeking behavior. However, these patients have not—as a rule—exhibited withdrawal symptoms, and the drug-seeking behavior may be motivated more by a wish to fool the physicians than by a desire for the drug itself.
- *Cerebral dysfunction:* A minority (perhaps 25%–30%) of Munchausen patients have evidence of cerebral dysfunction, with a greater verbal ability than logical or organizational ability. This

may facilitate pseudologia fantastica and its associated assumption of the patient role as an unconsciously motivated coping strategy.

- *Gratification of dependency needs:* Munchausen patients often have emotionally deprived backgrounds. Illness, with the requirement that someone else care for the sick person, is one way to have underlying dependency needs gratified. M. D. Feldman and Ford (1994) described this motivation as a search for nurturing.

- *Defense against psychosis:* Many Munchausen patients, by virtue of traumatic childhoods and a lack of mature coping mechanisms, are prone to acute anxiety that may overwhelm them and lead to a decline in reality testing. Such anxiety may be precipitated by a loss or by feelings of rejection or abandonment. The Munchausen behavior "organizes" the person. It establishes a role to be played, thereby creating a sense of identity. It turns a weak and helpless individual into a powerful, clever manipulator who is controlling the system. Simultaneously, the person's dependency needs (the search for nurturing) are met.

- *Need for identity:* Persons with Munchausen syndrome frequently have a poor sense of self. They have not created personal identities that define their value systems, goals, and roles in life. By simulating disease, they assume the well-defined role of sick persons, and through their pseudologia fantastica they become important and interesting patients. They are not ordinary, everyday patients; instead, they have rare, dramatic, or intriguing diseases. They present themselves as professional athletes, university presidents from foreign lands, or airline pilots. The constant quality of drama keeps them at center stage during their hospitalizations.

- *Need for mastery:* The Munchausen patient—who has a history of multiple emotional traumas, poor coping skills, a limited social support system, and poor occupational abilities—feels weak and vulnerable when not playing the Munchausen role. This weak, vulnerable feeling can be turned around through successful imposture of the patient role. Instead of feeling helpless, the Munchausen patient feels clever and powerful by fooling doctors and nurses (duping delight). The assumption of other roles (e.g., professional football player), which are believed by the hospital staff, provides the vicarious pleasure of being someone who is respected, important, and powerful. For example, one woman reported that she was an official of the World Health Organization who had the responsibility of caring for children displaced by war. Her story was believed by her health care providers, who openly admired her and spent extra time at her bedside providing supportive encouragement so that she could soon resume her important work for children in Southeast Asia.

▍ *Internalized anger or masochism:* One psychoanalytic interpretation for the patient's ready acceptance of the sick role, complete with painful or dangerous diagnostic and therapeutic procedures, is that there is underlying masochism (self-defeating behavior). Poor parenting, often involving physical or sexual abuse, may have resulted in a distorted self-image. This theory suggests that the anger directed toward the child has become internalized in the form of a devalued sense of the self as one who deserves nothing better than abuse. Because the limited attention received by the child was often associated with abuse, the Munchausen patient may consciously seek out situations (e.g., hospitalization) that mix nurturing (health care) with pain (surgical procedures). Incorporated into this formulation is the idea that a part (literally a part of the body) may need to be sacrificed to save the whole. It is the sense of self that must be preserved so that the person is not lost in a feeling of total emptiness.

The etiologies described above help us understand Stevie and Rose. Each was deprived as a child; each had a severe personality disorder that markedly restricted coping abilities; and each demonstrated Munchausen behavior in response to loss or rejection. Hospitalization gratifies underlying dependence needs, but these patients could simultaneously deny their needs and vulnerabilities by feeling superior to their caretakers (by virtue of having duped them). In this process, the patients devalued the caretakers (surrogates of the bad parents). It is noteworthy that the pseudologia fantastica produced by Rose was symbolic of the other losses and stressors in her life. She had indeed lost her parents and daughter, and she had been sexually abused; it was only the temporal relationships and the specific details that were incorrect.

Simple Factitious Disorder

Munchausen syndrome is the most extreme form of factitious disorder. There are milder forms of disease simulation that are determined by both conscious and unconscious motivations. Almost everyone has pleaded illness to avoid going to work or to avoid an unwanted social obligation (M. D. Feldman and Ford 1994). Other persons along this continuum may exhibit conversion disorders, somatization disorders, and hypochondriasis, all of which are presumably caused by unconscious factors. If there is some overt gain—such as avoiding military service or obtaining monetary awards from an insurance company—the deliberate simulation or production of disease is termed *malingering*. When the only apparent goal of the deliberate and surreptitious production of a disease is to play the sick role, the behavior is called *factitious disorder*.

Persons with simple, or nonperegrinating, factitious disorders are much more common than those with full-blown Munchausen syndrome. Typically, they do not use aliases and do not travel to cities away from their homes unless referred for consultation by their primary care physician. For example, a frustrated and confused primary care physician may refer such a patient to the Mayo Clinic because of difficulty in establishing a diagnosis or instituting effective treatment.

No one knows how frequently factitious behavior occurs, but it is believed to be much more common than recognized. For example, 3.5% of kidney stones submitted for pathological analysis proved to be of nonphysiological origin (Gault et al. 1988). Persons with simple factitious disorder have some of the psychological characteristics of Munchausen syndrome but in a less extreme manner. The following clinical case example illustrates simple factitious disorder.

■ The Anemic Nurse

The nurses on the hematology inpatient medical service all liked Janet. She was an attractive 34-year-old nurse who was hospitalized for a potentially fatal aplastic anemia. Janet's concerned mother and husband sat by her side daily, often helping monitor the rate of the intravenous infusions. She also received visitors from the nearby local hospital where she had worked as a nurse.

Janet's severe anemia remained unexplained but was presumed to be some type of autoimmune disease. She remained in semi-isolation for fear that even a minor infection might cause her death. Meanwhile, while hopefully waiting for her bone marrow to resume production of blood cells, Janet talked about her past life and mourned the loss of favorite activities such as horseback riding. She told of growing up on a farm where thoroughbreds were raised; she described taking her own horse from show to show in a trailer attached to her convertible in her teenage years, often accompanied by her wealthy, adoring, and indulgent father. After high school graduation, she had attended a prestigious West Coast university for a period of time, but she had decided that her vocation was caring for the sick and had returned home to attend nursing school. People's hearts went out to this glamorous patrician soul who might never recover from her life-threatening disease.

All of her caretakers' illusions were shattered when a test came back showing a blood level of methotrexate, a chemotherapeutic agent used for treating cancer. Subsequent investigation proved that Janet had been surreptitiously ingesting this drug and had knowingly caused her own severe anemia. This knowledge led to careful questioning of Janet's mother, who revealed that, contrary to Janet's story, her childhood experience had been one of a marginal financial existence after Janet's father deserted the family when she was a small child. Furthermore, her only higher education was at the local junior college. Before the acute onset of Janet's disease, her mother had become increasingly irritated and less accepting of Janet's demanding attitude. Janet's husband was a weak, ineffectual man who was also unable to meet her insatiable neediness.

Janet was genuinely very sick and, despite her ultimate recovery, could have died. She was a nurse, and she had to have complete understanding of her disease-producing behavior. Because she was not overtly suicidal, why did she do it? Janet's behavior was not as unusual as one might think. Factitious behavior, although not common, is not very rare and probably occurs much more frequently than is recognized.

Many of the possible psychological explanations for the behavior exhibited in Munchausen syndrome may also apply to the patient with simple factitious disorder. The need for nurturing may be a major component in determining the behavior. Many patients with factitious disorders are nurses or other caregivers. The disease allows a reversal of the usual role: instead of caring for someone else, they are now being cared for by others.

The case of Jenny described in the book on factitious disorders by M. D. Feldman and Ford (1994) illustrates the use of simulated disease to obtain nurturing. After an engagement was broken off, this patient disclosed to her co-workers that she had cancer. Her announcement was met with tremendous support and concern. Jenny kept the ruse active by deliberately losing weight and shaving her head to simulate the side effect of losing her hair from chemotherapy. She also joined a support group for cancer patients, but that proved to be her downfall because fellow group members recognized inconsistencies in her story. Friends and co-workers were predictably outraged when they learned of her fraudulent means of seeking emotional support.

Munchausen Syndrome by Proxy

The deliberate production of a disease in oneself is bizarre and difficult to comprehend. Unfortunately, extensive evidence indicates that some people deceptively produce disease in other people. This has become known as *Munchausen syndrome by proxy* (MSBP). The most common form of this syndrome is found in mothers who induce disease in their children or who falsely report symptoms that result in medical evaluations. The prevalence of MSBP is high enough to be recognized as a health hazard to children and has been defined as a form of child abuse. Hundreds, perhaps thousands, of cases have been reported to date (Schreier and Libow 1993).

A wide variety of diseases have been produced or simulated in children, usually in those of preverbal age. Methods of inducing symptoms may include smothering to the point of apnea, placing toxic substances in the mouths of infants, or falsely reporting symptoms such as seizures. In one case, a mother smeared catsup around the child's anus and told doctors that the child had rectal bleeding.

Once the child-victim has been hospitalized, the mother plays the role of the concerned, loving parent, always there, helpful and cooperative with the nurses. It has been proposed that by playing the role of the concerned mother of a sick child, the perpetrator becomes a central part of the drama and, as a result, receives support and care from others. MSBP is not a benign behavior. The mortality rate for these children (and their siblings) is in the range of 10% (Rosenberg 1987). Of importance, some of these mothers have previously engaged in factitious behaviors that involved their own bodies.

Another form of MSBP involves one adult inducing illness in another. One of the more abominable forms of this has been identified in nurses who surreptitiously cause acute medical emergencies, or even death, in patients under their care. A number of such situations have been reported, with many deaths being ascribed to single nurses (Yorker 1988). Various motivations have been offered to explain this heinous behavior. One of the more plausible, and consistent with parent-child MSBP, is that the nurses experience excitement and exhilaration when part of a cardiac arrest team: they are playing major roles in high drama.

Regardless of the various psychological motivations that may underlie MSBP, it is clear that the perpetrators are remarkably self-centered, nonempathetic, and unrespectful of the needs and rights of other persons. This pathological narcissism is also reflected in their use of deceit and lying. They make the world fit their own needs, even if blatant lying is required.

Summary

In this chapter, I have considered three categories of persons for whom deceiving others is a constant force in their lives: impostors, con artists, and persons who exhibit variations of Munchausen syndrome; all pretend to be something they are not. These three groups appear to share many characteristics. All appear to have significant impairment in their sense of personal identity and major difficulty establishing meaningful, warm, and intimate relationships with others. Their external personae are like movie sets—easily changed but with little substance behind the illusion created. Their predominant psychopathology is that generally characterized as narcissism. Because of a lack of empathy and defective interpersonal skills, they have not mastered mature, nonmanipulative ways to meet universal needs for nurturance, affection, and admiration. These deceivers are notably insensitive to the needs of other people, taking others' money, time, attention, and health, with little consideration or even awareness of the rights of other persons. They delight in their duping behavior because it gives them a sense of power or superiority as they devalue others.

Despite these similarities, there are also some differences. Con artists appear to have notable superego deficiencies and repeatedly engage in criminal activities. They more overtly "take" from others, and they are less dependent than the Munchausen patients, who "take" indirectly by assuming the sick role in order to manipulate others to care for them. Impostors who do not engage in illegal activities may be defending against depression and a sense of emptiness and inadequacy. Some impostors may even engage in altruistic activities as a part of their imposture. Persons with Munchausen syndrome (and its associated disorders) appear to be even more psychologically fragile than impostors, and they may use their behavior to defend against psychotic decompensation.

Those people described in this chapter are extraordinary. Most people will go through life without ever meeting an impostor, con artist, or person with one of the variations of Munchausen syndrome. Yet, as observed by Deutsch (1955), as we study these people, we see traces of them in the people with whom we interact every day and even in ourselves. An exaggerated form of these characteristics constitutes the material for motion pictures, but subtler forms are also common in people who do not pathologically lie. By studying the extreme examples, these subtle forms of living a lie become more identifiable in every person's construction of the personal myth.

Chapter 9

False Memories, False Accusations, and False Confessions

"I have done that," says my memory. "I cannot have done that," says my pride and remains adamant—at last memory yields.

—Nietzsche

Memory belongs to the imagination. Human memory is not like a computer which records things; it is part of the imaginative process, on the same terms as invention.

—Robbe-Grillet

The phenomenon of *recovered memories* is now attracting considerable interest in the United States. People are remembering events from their childhoods, events that include crimes of violence and sexual abuse. These memories, often recovered in psychotherapy, have led to painful disruptions of families, lawsuits, and even criminal prosecution. How do we examine this whole area of recovered memories in the context of lying? The issue of child abuse is so emotionally powerful that some have shied away from probing too deeply into the nature of recovered memories and psychotherapy. There has been increasing recognition of the importance of sexual abuse and harassment, yet we also know that distortions of memories can occur in psychotherapy as a result of the self-deceptions of the patient, the therapist, or both.

False accusations and false confessions of crimes also pose difficult questions about memory and truthfulness. Legal authorities face these falsehoods often. It is interesting to note that the areas of false memories, false accusations, and false confessions have many similarities.

In this chapter, I review basic concepts about memory and how its characteristics may affect the phenomena of recovered memories, false accusations, and false confessions. Knowledge about the nature of memory is of considerable practical importance in the conduct of psychotherapy, legal investigations, and courtroom testimony.

The Nature of Memory

Memory is what we are; if we lose our memories, we lose our identity and sense of self. As is the case with many other psychological phenomena, we think we know what memory is, yet when we examine it closely, its characteristics become elusive.

Our current views of how memory works divide it into three discrete processes: perception or registration, storage, and retrieval. Factors such as arousal, relation of information to the self, emotional state, and the intelligent filter influence perception (see Goleman 1985). The storage process is affected by the structural and physiological integrity of the brain. If there is bilateral loss of the hippocampus—that portion of the temporal lobes that is required for acquiring new information—then perceptions are not stored. Retrieval of memories is affected by one's emotional state, arousal, and current perceptions that stimulate associated memories.

This description of memory makes it sound like a personal computer with memories stored on the hard drive, awaiting the right program to call them up. Not quite! Although most of the general public and even many psychologists view memory as something that is fixed in the brain (like a computer file), research has shown that memory is continuously being reconstructed (Loftus and Loftus 1980). Old memories are updated with new perceptions, and prior memory traces are replaced. This process occurs outside of conscious awareness, and the individual does not perceive the new memory as new. This finding has enormous importance for the courtroom and the psychotherapist's office. The "old" memories that we so confidently treasure may, instead, be the recent suggestions of another person.

The evidence that individuals reconstruct memories instead of retaining fixed, permanent memories over time comes from both naturalistic observations and experimental work. Dr. Ulric Neisser, a psychologist at Emory University, conducted an experiment in which he asked a group of students the day after the *Challenger* space shuttle explosion where they were when they heard the news about the disaster. Two and a half years later, the same subjects were asked the same question. Even though all of the subjects vividly described their memories of the event, not one of the memories was entirely accurate, and one-third of the later descriptions were "wildly inaccurate" (Neisser and Harsch 1992). Other studies of eyewitness reports of dramatic events have demonstrated similar alterations in memory over time, even though the witnesses themselves are certain of the accuracy of their memories (Loftus and Ketcham 1994).

Experimental work by various investigators has yielded similar findings about the influence of later suggestions on a person's memory of an event. An example of this type of experiment is one conducted by Dr. Elizabeth Loftus of the University of Washington and her colleagues (Loftus and Hoffman 1989; Loftus et al. 1989a), in which subjects were shown a series of slides depicting a burglary. Then the subjects were exposed to differing narrative comments about the burglary, some of which contained misinformation (e.g., that the burglar used a hammer instead of a screwdriver). When the subjects were tested for their recall of details of the event, those who had been given misleading information after the original slide show were significantly more likely to misremember the details. The misled subjects were just as confident of the correctness of their answers as those who had not been misled. Furthermore, as judged by the reaction time of their answers (measured by the computer on which they were tested), the subjects felt no ambivalence about their responses. Loftus and her colleagues (1989b) concluded from this and similar experiments conducted in her laboratory, as well as from work by other scientists, that inaccurate memories can replace original memories in a manner that is not recognized by the person involved.

Our memories of past events are *not* like computer files but are highly malleable, fluid in time and space, and reflective of our current needs. Memories are being continuously reconstructed; the past is not fixed in memory. Rather, we remember the past in terms of our current emotions, experiences, and prejudices. For example, depressed people are much more likely to remember past negative events while they are depressed than they are when they recover from depression (Bower 1981). It is obvious that our memories of the past are distinctly influenced not only by our current emotional states but also by our relationships with others and what they may suggest to us, regardless of how subtle these suggestions may be (see section, "Courtroom Testimony," later in this chapter).

Recovered Memories

During the past decade, increased attention has been paid to childhood sexual and physical abuse. Many persons have come forward to state publicly that they were victims of such abuse during childhood. Some persons claim to have newly discovered knowledge of childhood abuse from "recovered memories."

■ The Jailed Granddaddy

It was early evening, and Herman, an elderly bespectacled gentleman already dressed in pajamas and bathrobe, responded to incessant knocking at his front door. Four policeman were on his doorstep, and one stepped forward and informed Herman that he was under arrest. After the mandatory reading of his rights, the frightened man was placed in the waiting police car and taken to the city jail. There, he was informed that his 38-year-old daughter, who lived in another state, had not only accused him of sexually abusing her as a child but also stated that he had abused her daughter during a recent vacation. Herman's wife arrived shortly thereafter with an attorney and bail bondsman and arranged his release. Until that night, Herman's prior "criminal" record was paying a magistrate $25 after being caught in the speed trap of a small southern Georgia town.

Herman had been married to the same woman for more than 40 years and had worked for almost the same length of time for a railroad company before his retirement 3 years before his arrest. He and his wife had sacrificed personal needs to send three children (including the accused daughter) to college. He had drunk an average of two beers per year (at the company picnic) and had attended his local church "every time the door opened." He professed, and his wife concurred, that he had enjoyed a satisfactory sexual relationship with her until quite recently, when his antihypertensive medication had caused some dysfunction. Herman's wife and two other children all, without question, denied the possibility of any sexual abuse. In fact, Herman's wife reported that Herman had never even been alone with his granddaughter during the vacation in which the alleged abuse had occurred.

The accusing daughter had been hospitalized twice during adolescence for depression. She was described as very bright but involved in a conflictive marriage. Recently, she had sought psychotherapy from a late-middle-aged male psychologist. He had used age-regression hypnotherapy as a treatment technique. The psychologist had helped her "recover" memories that extended back to when she was age 6 months, including memories of inappropriate sexual acts by her father. He also helped her "remember" events that demonstrated that her daughter, Herman's granddaughter, had been fondled.

Despite entreaties by multiple family members, the daughter remained adamant in maintaining her charges against her father. She was supported by her therapist, who stated that it was "not therapeutic for these things to be swept under the table." Meanwhile, Herman remained terrified that he would be extradited to another state and imprisoned by a kangaroo court.

The False Memory Syndrome Foundation. The story above is, unfortunately, characteristic of thousands of similar scenarios across the United States. Numerous magazine articles, professional journal reports, and books detail accounts of families being ripped apart, being impoverished by legal fees, and fearing criminal prosecution (Doe 1991; False Memory Syndrome Foundation 1994; "My Problem" 1994; Loftus 1993; Loftus and Ketcham 1994). Most individuals accused of perpetrating the abuse have maintained their innocence, but the accusing parties have been equally adamant in demanding justice. In one situation described by Loftus and Ketcham, a woman who had been sexually abused herself as a child and who had become a sexual abuse counselor found herself accused of perpetrating sexual abuse. She was eventually cleared of the charges but not before she was fired from her job.

Counseling for sexual abuse has become a thriving cottage industry. All over the United States, there are now therapists whose expertise in recovered memories may be limited to owning a copy of *The Courage to Heal* (Bass and Davis 1988, 1994), a bestselling "Guide for Women Survivors of Child Sexual Abuse," currently in its third edition. These sexual abuse counselors are identifying and treating women (and a few men) who in the course of therapy "remember" being sexually abused during childhood. Many of these cases consist of persons who "recovered" their memories during therapy, like Herman's daughter. Tens of thousands of people are involved in this epidemic. In response to this onslaught, a group of persons who claim to have been unfairly accused have banded together to form the False Memory Syndrome Foundation (FMSF), the scientific and professional board of which is composed of many distinguished psychologists and psychiatrists.

FMSF is a nonprofit organization dedicated to providing group support to those who claim to have been falsely accused and to encouraging scientific research of the false memory syndrome (FMSF 1994). As of October 1994, FMSF has on file more than 14,000 reports that fit the false memory syndrome pattern. About 300 of the accusers later recanted their accusations.

Dr. Paul R. McHugh, professor of psychiatry and chairman of the department of psychiatry and behavioral sciences at Johns Hopkins University, is a member of the advisory board of the FMSF. He has compared the current epidemic of multiple personality disorder with its putative causes in childhood sexual abuse to the Salem witch hunts of the seventeenth century (McHugh 1992). He has observed that some psychiatrists/psychologists frequently make the diagnosis of multiple personality disorder after suggesting the symptoms to suggestible patients. These same clinicians, in accordance with their preconceived theories as to the etiology of multiple personality disorder, find memories of sexual abuse. Thus, both the illness and its supposed etiology are of iatrogenic origins. Dr. McHugh has called for greater science and less hysteria in our psychiatric evaluation of patients (McHugh 1994).

Assisted by data collected in conjunction with FMSF, Wakefield and Underwager (1992) compiled information about the typical accuser and the typical therapist. The accusing adults were 90% female, were mostly college educated, and typically came from intact, functional, and successful families. Only about one-third of these women had received psychiatric treatment during their childhood or adolescence.

The common trait of these accusers was that they had received therapy. Almost all "memories" were "recovered" during psychotherapy that had often included hypnotherapy, dream interpretation, and survivor groups. In almost all cases, *The Courage to Heal* was used along with other survivor or self-help books (see below). Seventy-five percent of the therapists were female, and most were psychologists, counselors, or social workers; only 8% were psychiatrists. More than half of the female therapists were between ages 30 and 39.

Incest survivor books.   Several self-help books are currently available for the woman who was, or thinks she may have been, abused as a child. *The Courage to Heal* (Bass and Davis 1988, 1994) is regarded as the "bible" of these books. As of January 1993, it had sold more than 500,000 copies. *The Courage to Heal* openly encourages its women readers to believe that they have been abused. Several common nonspecific symptoms (including low self-esteem, trouble feeling motivated, or a proneness to depression) are listed as typical of a postabuse syndrome. Furthermore, the book suggests that if a woman thinks she might have been abused, then she almost certainly was. (In the face of severe criticism, this suggestion was slightly toned down in the 1994 revised edition of the book.)

Carol Tavris, writing in the *New York Times Book Review* (1993), commented that the incest survivor books contain fabricated statistics; no empirical data support the high frequency of sexual abuse that they report. She went on to observe that the books are frequently countertherapeutic. She stated that "contemporary incest survivor books encourage women to incorporate the language of victimization and survival into the sole organizing narrative of their identity. It becomes their major story. . . . There can be little doubt that these incest survival books serve to help create new victims, to expand the market for the role of more books, and to necessitate the need for therapy" (Tavris 1993, p. 17).

Accurate data for the incidence of childhood sexual abuse in the general population are not available. The prevalence of reports of remembered sexual abuse is notably high in some selected populations, such as women with psychiatric diagnoses, particularly borderline personality disorder, eating disorders, and somatization disorder. From anecdotal information, there can be little doubt that genuine sexual abuse is common and a major cause of psychological distress. The issue is not whether sexual abuse occurs but whether all claims of sexual abuse are true.

Implantation of false memories. The epidemic of "recovered" memories appears to be related to women having seen certain psychotherapists or to reading self-help books about childhood sexual abuse. If this is the situation, and many of the recovered memories are indeed false, how is the phenomenon to be explained?

George K. Ganaway, a psychiatrist in Atlanta, has provided some interesting and plausible hypotheses as to why persons may remember something that never happened. He reported that patients who described improbable memories of satanic ritual abuse were often persons with borderline and narcissistic personality disorders and who demonstrated a high degree of hypnotizability (suggestibility) and a proneness to fantasy (Ganaway 1989). Ganaway suggested that these patients may be reacting to subtle suggestions from the therapist. They use these fantasies (which become memory) to create a screen that blocks out consideration of other areas of genuine distress in their lives. In this process, the patients create an inaccurate narrative of their lives. This reconstruction of one's life may significantly, but temporarily, reduce acute distress and anxiety by offering seemingly logical explanations for one's unhappiness. Furthermore, through this process the person may, as a consequence of the disclosure of "remembered abuse," receive support from the therapist as well as from survivor groups and from self-identification with the survivor movement (Ganaway 1994).

The deliberate implantation of false memories appears to be much easier than one might think. Loftus and Ketcham (1994) reported that they had assigned students to attempt to induce false memories in an acquaintance or relative. All students found it relatively easy to induce memories such as getting lost at a shopping mall, when the actual event never occurred. The techniques used were very simple and included asking questions such as "Do you remember the time you got lost at the mall?" In fact, some of the subjects of these homegrown experiments quickly elaborated on and increased the extent of their own false memories.

Accuracy of recovered memories. There is no doubt that sexual abuse and physical violence do occur in the lives of children, but two questions must be asked: 1) To what extent are the memories of abuse repressed? 2) When a memory of childhood is recovered during adulthood, how accurate is that memory? Some psychologists do not endorse the idea of repression and hence would be skeptical of any recovered memory. Others believe that a single traumatic event may be repressed (dissociated from consciousness), but it is unlikely that a series of repeated traumas occurring over time would be completely repressed (Loftus 1993). Of those psychologists and psychiatrists who do believe that childhood trauma can be repressed, some tend to accept unquestioningly the veracity of these memories, and some believe that memories can be either accurate (in spirit if not in exact detail) or false.

In some cases, people have been convicted of murder decades after the crime because of evidence presented through recovered memories (Appelbaum 1992). Recovered memories of violent crimes are rare, but criminal and civil legal proceedings for alleged sexual abuse, based on recovered memories, are becoming more common. These proceedings, when based on false memories, can destroy the lives of innocent people. Gutheil (1993) and Appelbaum (1992) emphasized the differences between accepting a patient's statements as "narrative truth" in psychotherapy and claiming "historical truth" in the courtroom. The level of certainty that an event actually occurred must be much greater for the latter than the former. Gutheil also stated that the therapist who recovers such memories may be a witness of fact but that the court should not recognize the therapist as an expert; such a dual role is unethical because the court has an egalitarian obligation to protect both plaintiff and defendant.

It is indisputable that some victims of true abuse have belatedly come forth to press genuine grievances. How does a professional, who was not present at the time of the alleged abuse, make an assessment of the likelihood of such abuse? Obviously, absolute proof is rarely available. Wakefield and Underwager (1992) have listed a number of issues for therapists who encounter the phenomenon of recovered memory to consider:

- All prior and current medical, psychiatric, and school records for the person claiming abuse should be obtained and reviewed.
- Information about the past and present interpersonal relationships of the person who claims to have been abused should be obtained; direct interviews with these persons, especially relatives such as siblings, are exceedingly valuable.
- A complete sexual history of the person who claims to have been abused should be obtained.
- The manner in which the information about the abuse was obtained must be determined. Was it during age-regression hypnosis, or did the treating therapist ask leading questions? Did the information emerge during a survivors' group meeting? Contrary to the views of many psychotherapists (Yapko 1994), information obtained under hypnosis is not reliable (Council on Scientific Affairs 1985).
- Whether the accusations emerged during therapy with a counselor or therapist who frequently "discovers" evidence of sexual abuse among his or her clients should be determined.
- The accusing individual's exposure to books (e.g., *The Courage to Heal*), workshops, or television shows about sexual abuse should be established.
- Recent stresses or evidence of psychiatric illness in the accusing individual should be evaluated.

▌ Whether the memories reported include blatantly improbable reports of satanic cult abuse, cannibalism, and similar activities should be examined (Ganaway 1989).

▌ Whether the characteristics of the reported memories are clearly inconsistent with the known physiological properties of memory should be investigated. For example, memories of events before age 3½ years are very improbable, and memories before age 2 years are essentially impossible (Loftus et al. 1994; Usher and Neisser 1993).

▌ The psychological characteristics (e.g., stability, alcoholism) of the family of origin in which the alleged events occurred should be evaluated.

▌ Whether the accuser previously made other accusations, such as sexual harassment by co-workers or supervisors, should be assessed.

▌ Any evidence of prior criminal behavior in the accused person that would support or undermine the credibility of the allegations should be analyzed.

▌ Any personal records, pornographic photographs, or other evidence (such as statements by siblings, relatives, or childhood friends) that would support the allegations should be investigated.

▌ Any suggestion that the accuser may receive benefit or reinforcement from the allegations (e.g., acceptance by members of a group, monetary gain from a lawsuit, or rationalization for personal failures) should be explored.

▌ Whether resistance or refusal by the person making the accusation or the accuser's therapist to seek a second opinion from a respected authority in psychology or psychiatry exists should be determined.

None of the information related to the above issues (with the exception of concrete evidence such as photographs) definitely establishes or refutes the accuracy of recovered memories. However, clear patterns suggest the probability or improbability of the allegations. Therapists and expert witnesses in such cases are advised to consider all of the potential evidence carefully.

Many sexual abuse counselors are sincere in their beliefs and wishes to help people whom they perceive as victims. However, when large sums of money and people's livelihoods are involved, one cannot resist the cynical observation that the continuing discovery of "recovered memories" is big business to both therapists and booksellers.

Memory, Deception, and Psychotherapy

In 1994, a southern California jury, after hearing the evidence, agreed with Gary Ramona that a psychiatrist and counselor had acted improperly by inducing false memories of sexual abuse in his daughter (Grinfeld 1994). Ramona was awarded $500,000, despite the fact that his daughter continued to insist that her memories were true. He later settled out of court for less, in exchange for the defendant's agreement not to appeal. Because of the settlement, there will be no appellate review and, therefore, no precedent set by a higher court. In a similar case, a Dallas jury awarded $500,000 to a couple, saying that a psychiatrist had slandered them by falsely accusing them of sexually abusing their now-grown daughter (S. J. Brown 1995). It is likely that these cases have long-standing implications for the liability of psychotherapists. They set a precedent that a third party can be injured by psychotherapy, and this third party can successfully seek redress for the wrongdoing.

These two cases are similar to other situations described in this book. Although sexual abuse and murder are dramatic criminal acts, other forms of "recovered memories" may be equally insidious in their damage. How many persons, during and after psychotherapy, have accused parents and spouses of a variety of less dramatic forms of abuse? How many times has psychotherapy led to the decision to divorce a bewildered spouse? Statistics are not available, but, anecdotally, persons working in the mental health field know that such an outcome is not uncommon. Frequently used explanations (rationalizations) include the contention that the abandoned spouse did not "grow" with the one in psychotherapy or that psychotherapy helped a person gain the courage to get out of an unhappy marriage. These reasons may apply to some situations, but another explanation is that a person may develop misperceptions, which become his or her "truth," during the process of psychotherapy.

The patient in psychotherapy must be selective about which information in his or her life to bring to the therapy session. There are automatic biases of retrospection, in that memory traces are influenced by beliefs and feelings in the present. As noted by Dawes (1988), we "literally 'make up stories' about our lives, the world, and reality in general . . . and often . . . it is the story that creates the memory, rather than vice versa" (p. 107). The patient's story, as it unfolds in psychotherapy, is also markedly influenced by the process of transference (feelings toward, and ideas about, the therapist). Thus, with the patient's tendency to choose which areas to discuss (and which to ignore), the patient's life story can be guided by the therapist, by both overt statements and subtle messages. As the story is told and retold (similar to "thought reform" described later in this chapter), it becomes increasingly accepted as fact; the story *becomes* the patient's memory and the patient's reality.

As a consequence of the creation of a new life story, problems may be externalized. The person's internal pain may be blamed on others because of sexual or physical abuse in the past, an unsympathetic spouse, self-centered parents, or the sexism or racism of society. Although sexism and racism are very real and cause significant pain among those who experience such discrimination, some people may use these factors as a scapegoat to explain their distress and shortcomings. This process may be temporarily comforting, but it may also, as noted by Tavris (1993), serve as a screen to hide the real problems and life's real pain from the individual.

Our increasing understanding of the nature of memory and the subtle ways in which it can be influenced (see section, "Courtroom Testimony," below) forces us to take a new look at the process of psychotherapy and to be more aware of the importance of the therapist's input during psychotherapy (Bonanno 1990).

Therapists may knowingly or unknowingly participate in the process of creating a new narrative truth. Among the ways that a therapist's own issues may be displaced into the therapy are strongly held political biases (e.g., the belief that all women's problems are caused by exploitation of women in a male-dominated society); theoretical biases (e.g., the belief that the primary cause for multiple personality disorder or eating disorders is childhood sexual abuse); internal or interpersonal conflicts (e.g., the therapist's sexual or marital conflicts being projected into the therapy); or conscious greed (e.g., creating new victims of sexual abuse in order to provide services for them). It is increasingly obvious that the therapist's biases may be incorporated into a patient's memory.

Psychotherapy has enormous power, both to heal and—like any potent therapeutic intervention—to harm (Strupp et al. 1977). Psychotherapy, unfortunately, is often conducted by persons who have little training. In other situations, psychotherapists who are ostensibly well trained may rely on feelings for evidence, on metaphors for reality, and on inspiration and myth for guidance, instead of using empirical knowledge (McHugh 1994). In my opinion, psychotherapy is more likely to be beneficial when several of the conditions below are fulfilled. These somewhat provocative suggestions are based on increasing scientific knowledge of the malleability of memory and on personal or professional experience of situations in which psychotherapy proved harmful to the patient or to third parties.

- The traditional view that it is only the patient's perceptions that are important (i.e., that historical accuracy is not important) must be reexamined. Instead, increased emphasis must be placed on bringing significant other persons into the therapy. Such an approach will minimize, but not eliminate, the induction of false memories.

- The importance of maintaining therapeutic neutrality cannot be overemphasized. The therapist's political views, theoretical perspectives, personal emotions and problems, and opinions should intrude as little as possible into the therapy. Furthermore, as emphasized by Ganaway (1989), in the absence of independent corroboration, the therapist should maintain a neutral attitude concerning the veracity of the patient's reports of the present, the past, and of other people's actions.

- Hypnosis or similar regressive techniques should never be employed by anyone who does not have extensive training in its limitations, applications, implications, and contraindications.

- Therapists who provide insight-oriented (reconstructive) psychotherapy, or variations thereof, must receive extensive supervised training that includes an emphasis on understanding the power of transference, the risks of countertransference, and the nature of memory.[1] Many therapists who consider themselves "experts" are actually deceiving themselves by failing to recognize their limitations in providing this form of psychotherapy. The problem is akin to a physician who was trained to perform simple surgical procedures but assumes that he or she can do heart transplants.

■ The importance of the risk that the therapist's own personal beliefs, feelings, and conflicts can be injected into psychotherapy must be recognized. Personal psychotherapy for the therapist, or very closely supervised work during training, will reduce but not eliminate this risk.

■ Second opinions, now common for medical or surgical procedures, may be even more valuable for patients who are in, or about to start, intensive psychotherapy.

In summary, the deceptions and self-deceptions of both patient and therapist may markedly influence the course and outcome of psychotherapy. The importance of the malleability of memory cannot be overemphasized. Although dramatic accusations of recovered memories of childhood sexual abuse have garnered the spotlight, other distortions of memory, resulting from a breakdown of the therapist's neutrality, are also frighteningly common in psychotherapy. Furthermore, it is not only the patient but also third parties who are at risk from the damage caused by misadventures in psychotherapy.

---

[1] *Insight-oriented psychotherapy* is based on psychoanalytic theory and techniques. The goal of this form of therapy is to create beneficial changes by increasing the patient's understanding of his or her unconscious mental processes. During therapy, the patient may experience *transference,* that is, feelings or ideas toward the therapist that are reenactments of similar feelings toward people in the patient's past. For example, a patient who was repeatedly criticized by a parent might feel that the therapist is critical and respond accordingly. Therapists may also have inappropriate emotional reactions to patients, a phenomenon called *countertransference.* For example, a therapist whose childhood was marked by intense sibling rivalry might display competitive feelings and behaviors toward a professionally successful patient.

The patient who seeks psychotherapy almost invariably requests help in modifying feelings, behaviors, or thoughts that are personally uncomfortable. In another situation—*thought reform*—the individual may be an involuntary party in the effort to produce psychological changes.

Thought Reform (Brainwashing)

We can examine historical events to gain a better understanding of the implantation of false memories that has led to false confessions. During the mid-1950s, there was considerable interest in the reported efforts of communists, both in the Soviet Union and communist Asia, to "brainwash" political prisoners. There was an apparent effort to change the beliefs (and memories) of these persons, not just to punish them as was done with common criminals (Berle 1957). Prisoners of war (POWs) were considered to be enemies of the state and, therefore, were also subject to thought-reform techniques. Americans who were captured during the Korean War (1950–1953) and the captured *Pueblo* crew members (1967–1968) reported that the North Koreans made efforts to influence their beliefs. For the *Pueblo* crew, this influence was largely extended though efforts to coerce confessions and to "educate" them through lectures and demonstrations (Ford 1975). Some of the American POWs in the Korean War were subjected to much more intensive efforts at thought reform, and a few refused to be repatriated, presumptive evidence of success in changing their beliefs (Segal 1954).

The communist police and other authorities involved in the thought-reform process used fairly simple techniques (Biderman 1957; Hinkle and Wolff 1956, 1957; Lifton 1957; Segal 1954). The prisoner was made susceptible to thought reform by enforced isolation, degradation, and threats in order to cause fear, regression, and increased suggestibility. At the point of the prisoner's loss of psychological equilibrium and need for rescue, there was a shift to a different approach: calculated leniency. The interrogator, perhaps a new person, was introduced to the victim, who at this time had an intense need for human contact and would therefore see the interrogator as a potential rescuer. An important component of thought reform was the alternating production of tension followed by release of tension through approval and acceptance. The victim was required to make a "confession," often in the form of a long written account of his or her personal history. The thought reformer reviewed this history with the victim and may have vaguely provided a little praise here and there but in an ambiguous manner that indicated that the history was unsatisfactory. This process was repeated many times, and the history evolved. The victim often felt considerable relief when the history was approved. The victims' personal histories as recorded on paper and in memories were progressively altered to meet the needs of the perpetrator. These new memories, which were presented as confessions, were a complex blend of rationalizations, altered memories, and confabulations.

The Chinese and North Koreans made greater use of group process as a means to effect thought reform. The groups consisted of six to eight prisoners crowded in a small cell. This setting exploited the emotional nakedness and sense of unworthiness that the self-criticism techniques generated in the prisoners through the repetitious rewriting of their autobiographies. These groups generated enormous pressures for conformity (see "Groupthink," Chapter 13) and thereby markedly reinforced the process of thought reform. Hinkle and Wolff (1956) reported that "the ultimate achievement of a proper rationalization and group acceptance is associated with feelings of relief that are occasionally exhilarating, and sometimes show some of the features of a religious 'conversion'" (p. 174). Another reinforcement for thought reform was the use of selected reading materials.

This description of thought reform bears more than a faint resemblance to some forms of psychotherapy, particularly to some of those types of counseling that have led to recovered memories. A patient, already in distress, may go to a therapist who repeatedly asks him or her to describe childhood experiences. "Memories" of past sexual abuse or other life problems are differentially reinforced. In addition, the patient's "new understanding" of the cause for his or her distress can be further reinforced through group experiences and outside readings. Hinkle and Wolff's comment about the features of a religious "conversion" are often appropriate for these situations.

False Accusations

The contemporary media frequently report situations in which dramatic accusations have been made by a victim and are alleged to be false by the accused person. These accusations often involve sexual harassment or sexual abuse. Many of these accusations are firmly rooted in reality; some are false.

■ The Rape Victim

A 49-year-old married woman, who claimed to have been raped in the dressing room of a nationally known department store, garnered national publicity and sympathy (Jones 1993). She had emerged from the dressing room partially clothed and disheveled and stated that she had been raped. Examination disclosed superficial vaginal abrasions and semen on her clothing. A reward for information leading to the conviction of the perpetrator was offered by the department store, which had been criticized for lax security. The police department held a news conference to ask for public assistance in locating the rapist. In fact, she had not been raped. A careful investigation indicated that the woman had inflicted the wounds on herself with duct tape and sprinkled herself with a vial of her husband's semen. For unspecified reasons, neither the department store nor the police department pressed charges, and the anonymity of the false victim was maintained.

False accusations are a vicious form of lie, one of the most aggressive verbal assaults that can occur. False allegations of sexual assault may be among the more common forms of this type of lie. National attention has recently been directed toward sexual abuse, and many such allegations have emerged. Many allegations are true, but some are false (Matas and Marriott 1987). Such false allegations are not a recent phenomenon; Healy and Healy (1915), in their classic book published 80 years ago, described many instances of false accusations of sexual abuse and assaults. Other authors have described similar cases (Dohn 1986; M. D. Feldman and Ford 1994; Matas and Marriott 1987; S. Snyder 1986; Soules et al. 1978).

One motivation of the individual reporting the assault may be to attack a man for perceived wrongs. This obvious motivation may, however, be relatively infrequent or less important than are the "victim's" intrapsychic needs. The accusations may be a projection onto others of a woman's own angry, aggressive, internally disordered psyche and ambivalence about her own sexuality (S. Snyder 1986). Another motivation may be the need to play the role of the victim. In this situation, the accused perpetrator is just an ancillary prop. As a victim, the woman becomes the center of attention, concern, sympathy, and nurturing care. In many ways, these accusers resemble patients with other factitious disorders (see Chapter 8). Like such patients, most of the women who falsely claim that they were raped meet the descriptive criteria for histrionic or borderline personality disorder.

False Confessions

At the opposite end of the phenomenological spectrum from those who make false accusations are people who confess to crimes they did not commit. Both categories of individuals share a tendency toward pathological lying.

■ The Hanged Liar

Timothy Evans was eventually granted a royal pardon, but the pardon came years after he was hanged in 1950 for a murder that he did not commit (Sharrock and Cresswell 1989). Evans had initially presented himself at a police station, where he confessed to having murdered his wife and daughter. He subsequently made a series of inconsistent confessions that he later retracted. He was convicted by a jury because of the initial confession, which (because he was a known liar) superseded in the jury's mind his subsequent retractions. He was described by his mother as having a vivid imagination and being a "terrible liar." Of note, he was also of below-average intelligence and was barely able to read.

Several similarities exist between Evans and another Englishman who falsely confessed to a murder. This man styled himself as "Lord A., the fifth Marquis of Bath" (a bogus title) and also engaged in other pseudologia fantastica. (For a discussion of pseudologia fantastica, see Chapters 2 and 7.) He was studied by Sharrock and Cresswell (1989), who found that he was of average intelligence but had dyslexia and other nonspecific neuropsychological dysfunctions. He was also found to be extroverted, highly suggestible, and compliant to interpersonal pressure.

Dr. Gisli Gudjonsson of London has studied a large number of persons who have allegedly made false confessions. Gudjonsson found that when these persons were compared with other persons referred for forensic evaluations, those with supposedly false confessions were notably less intelligent and more suggestible and compliant (Gudjonsson 1990). Caution must be exercised in evaluating any confession and the means by which it was obtained. Factors shown to influence a person to make a false confession include being kept in custody for an extended time with no access to lawyers, friends, or family; lack of control over the physical environment; being subordinate to a powerful legitimate authority; inadequate food and sleep; intimidation by police officers; and being fearful for one's personal safety (Gudjonsson and MacKeith 1988). These factors are also consistent with the thought-reform techniques used to obtain false confessions from political prisoners.

Law enforcement officers are well aware of the phenomenon of multiple spontaneously generated false confessions following a highly publicized crime. Such a confession may reflect an individual's need for attention (no matter how such attention is obtained) or difficulty in distinguishing reality from fantasy, especially in a guilt-ridden person.

Courtroom Testimony

Two sincere witnesses can provide diametrically opposed testimony in a court of law, each believing that he or she is telling the truth and that the other is lying. Tragically, many innocent persons have been falsely convicted, imprisoned, and even sentenced to death on the basis of faulty eyewitness testimony (Loftus and Ketcham 1991). The concepts of the malleability of memory help us to understand how differently people can perceive and remember an event.

Furthermore, we have learned how the memory of an event can be manipulated by another person by the use of postevent suggestions.

Leading questions by investigators, police officers, attorneys, or even psychotherapists can also markedly and permanently alter a person's memory. Loftus and Palmer (1974) demonstrated that by altering the wording of a question, they also could alter a person's recollection of an event. These researchers had subjects view a videotape that showed two cars colliding with each other and asked the subjects to estimate the speed at which the cars were traveling. When the question was phrased, "How fast were the cars going when they *smashed* into each other?" subjects judged the speed to be significantly higher than when the question was phrased, "How fast were the cars going when they *hit* each other?" One week later, the same subjects were asked if they had seen broken glass at the scene of the accident (no glass had been present). Subjects who had been asked the "smashed" question were more likely to say "yes" than those who had been asked the "hit" question (Loftus 1975). Thus, there was an elaboration of memory that extended beyond the wording of the initial simple question. Furthermore, a very subtle difference in a question could yield different answers. Subjects who were asked, "Did you see *the* broken headlight?" were more likely to answer "yes" than those who were asked, "Did you see *a* broken headlight?" (Loftus and Zanni 1975).

Loftus has interpreted (and I certainly agree) the findings of her research as indicating that how witnesses are interrogated by the police, prepared by an attorney, and examined on the witness stand can all significantly influence their testimony. Someone else's ideas can easily become a part of an individual's memory and testimony under oath.

Controversy surrounds the reliability of children's memories and their competency to provide accurate testimony in court. Research studies such as those by Ceci and colleagues (1987) and Tate and colleagues (1992) indicate that children as young as age 3 or 4 years do "lie" or "misremember" and that they are more likely to do so in response to suggestions made by an authority figure with whom they are familiar. From their research, and consistent with research performed with adults, Ceci and colleagues found that "post-event suggestions can in fact distort memory" (p. 38).

Research conducted by Haugaard (1993) found that small children, including preschoolers, have an accurate concept of what constitutes a lie. Essentially all children understand the difference between the truth and a lie by the time they are in first grade. However, their memories can become distorted when the authority of an adult corroborates a lie. Haugaard's research technique involved using a videotape in which the "facts" were clear. In one version of the tape, a boy lied to a man that his daughter had hit the boy while the boy's mother passively listened. All of the children clearly recognized the lie. In another version, the mother actively lied in support of the boy's lies to the man. In the latter version, the children's memories of what had actually happened were distorted, and preschoolers and kindergarten children in particular were more likely to remember that one child had hit another when, in fact, that had not occurred.

A recent scholarly review by Ceci and Bruck (1993) synthesized the empirical data available concerning the suggestibility of child witnesses. These authors concluded that children—even preschoolers—are capable of recalling information that is forensically relevant. They also cautioned that children are suggestible (as are adults) and that how they are interrogated may influence their memories of events. Children are more likely to "recall" events that have been suggested to them if interrogated repetitively with leading questions. Just like adults, children may shape their memories and testimony to conform with the wishes of an authority figure.

Summary

Memory, on close examination, proves to be far more malleable than is generally recognized. A person's recollection of an event is in a process of continual reconstruction, influenced by the personal relevance of new information, emotions, and current stimuli. Important among these influences are the suggestions of other people. Friends, acquaintances, police officers, attorneys, or psychotherapists can—by suggestion or leading questions—create new and confidently held memories in other people. This effect is enhanced if the person making the suggestion is perceived as an authority figure. Patients in psychotherapy may construct an inaccurate past. People who were eyewitnesses to a crime may remember things that never occurred, and individuals may confess to crimes that they did not commit. An angry woman may falsely accuse a man of rape and then, after many repetitions, come to believe her own story. Political views and a specified view of history may be systematically foisted on a political prisoner, who is "reformed" in the process.

The bottom line is that one person's self-deceptions or overt lies can become another person's firmly held memories and "truth."

Chapter 10

Detection of Deceit

He who has eyes to see and ears to hear may convince
himself that no mortal can keep a secret. If his lips are
silent, he chatters with his fingertips: betrayal oozes out
of him at every pore.

—Freud

We live in the information age, inundated with a constant flood of data. Not only are we always receiving information from interactions with other people, the truth of which must be continually evaluated, but we must also sift through a seemingly limitless flow of information from the media—the press, radio, television, and even our computer modems. If information is power—and that is certainly the message from both philosophers and government policymakers—then misinformation decreases power. Thus, we must all be lie detectors, continuously expending energy to evaluate the input of information for its validity and for the motivation of its sender.

There seem to be socially acceptable standards for seeking out the truth. If an individual is too accepting and unquestioning of information, we call that person gullible or unsophisticated. If an individual is too vigilant and suspicious, we call that person paranoid. There appears to be an optimal range of deceit-detection activity, and some acceptance of information without too much

197

question is regarded as socially appropriate.

In this chapter, I focus on the lie detection that everyone practices on a daily basis. In Chapter 11, I address technological methods of detecting deceit.

Humans as Lie Detectors

A 14-year-old boy stands before his high school principal, accused of stealing another boy's watch from a locker. The boy stammers and denies the charges, leans on one foot and then the other, and stares at the bookcase rather than looking at the principal. The principal does not know that the boy has a domineering, abusive father who frequently beats him for perceived misbehaviors. How is the principal likely to assess the truthfulness of the boy's denial, and what action is the principal likely to initiate?

We all expend a considerable amount of psychic energy evaluating the constant input of new information. This information is checked against previously acquired knowledge, and older information is reevaluated in light of new data. This process is so automatic that it usually goes unnoticed, reaching consciousness only when there are major discrepancies or when disturbing emotions are elicited. Because of our need for self-deception, we frequently choose not to consciously challenge false information, either new or old. However, much of the new input and its evaluation may be registered unconsciously, having subsequent effects on our emotions and behaviors.

A clinical example that illustrates the effect of unconsciously registered inconsistent information was the onset of panic attacks in a young man who was on vacation with his parents. He had not experienced any apparent stressful precipitating events, but when he returned home, he learned that his girlfriend had been sexually unfaithful to him. During subsequent psychiatric evaluation, it was apparent to both the psychiatrist and the young man that the girlfriend had been deceiving him for some weeks. He had unconsciously registered data that indicated betrayal, but because it was incompatible with his desire to be loved and his need to maintain the relationship, he had not allowed this unacceptable information to reach consciousness. Yet, at a time when the girlfriend was acting out her infidelity (with the opportunity presented by the vacation), he had responded with severe anxiety, the cause for which he did not recognize at the time. Similarly, another patient's panic attacks began during separation from his lover during a business trip. The symptoms preceded conscious acknowledgment that the relationship was in trouble and the conscious knowledge of the lover's promiscuous behavior.

Regardless of our conscious intent, as humans, we are constantly evaluating the validity of the information we receive. Because words alone may be difficult to challenge, we use other means to check the "truthfulness" of the message we receive. In face-to-face or vocal encounters (e.g., the telephone), we rely heavily on the help of nonverbal communication. To do this, we rapidly process large amounts of different types of data and reach an "intuitive" conclusion about whether a person is lying. Relatively few people deliberately and consciously break this mass of data down into separate components.

In any one message, there are many forms of communication. I individually describe each of these "channels," keeping in mind that many channels are usually involved in any one message and that they often operate simultaneously. The communication includes the words themselves; the cadence, volume, and pitch of the voice; facial expressions; movements or posturing of the trunk and limbs; and observable physiological reactions to emotion, such as flushed cheeks or sweaty hands.

Much of the scientific work that elucidates nonverbal communications and their relation to deceit was pioneered by Paul Ekman and his co-workers (1969b) at the Langley Porter Psychiatric Institute of the University of California, San Francisco. Others who have significantly contributed to our understanding of nonverbal communications and deceit include Bella DePaulo and her co-workers at the University of Virginia, Robert Feldman at Harvard University, and Miron Zuckerman at the University of Rochester.

One hypothesis suggests that when a person is attempting to deceive, he or she is more cognitively challenged, guilty, anxious, or insecure than a person who is telling the truth (B. M. DePaulo et al. 1985a). Physiological changes occur in association with increased emotion, and the person may also demonstrate behavioral changes that can be detected by others. The emotional changes (e.g., anxiety) can be fueled by the discussion of the topic itself (regardless of the truthfulness of what is being said), fear of the consequences of not being believed, or guilt about a behavior that is considered to be wrong or sinful. Thus, emotional activation is more likely to occur when the topic is conflictive or emotionally arousing. Such a discussion might involve anger or sexual issues. Furthermore, there may be more arousal when the stakes are high (e.g., if the liar will be punished if he or she is not believed). A person who believes that deceit is sinful may become very guilty when lying, showing fear or anxiety, even though the lie may be morally justified (e.g., a lie to the Gestapo about the whereabouts of Jews in hiding).

On the other hand, a person telling the truth may have increased emotional arousal in some of these same situations. There may be fears that the truth is not recognized, or the topic under discussion may be conflictive or embarrassing. Furthermore, not everyone demonstrates emotion and discomfort in the same manner or to the same degree, even under similar circumstances. Ekman (1992) has used the term *Othello error* to illustrate the risk of misinterpreting emotional response as evidence of lying. He has also used the term *idiosyncratic error* to describe situations in which a person may have some personal characteristic behaviors that others may regard as evidence of deceit. For example, some people characteristically have little eye contact with those to whom they are speaking. Such an individual may be regarded as lying, when this behavior actually has no relation to the content or veracity of the communication.

Another potential error in assessing a person's truthfulness based on emotional arousal is the possibility that not everyone reacts physiologically to apparent anxiety-provoking situations. Individuals with antisocial personalities, the very people most likely to lie perniciously, appear to have lower levels of autonomic and subjective anxiety in social situations (Lykken 1957; Schmauk 1970). Ironically, the very people in whom one may wish to detect deception may be the most difficult to decipher.

Nonverbal Clues to Deceit

Several investigators have used different research techniques to determine which verbal, behavioral, and physiological responses are most characteristic of lying. Experimental subjects may be asked to talk about someone, providing their truthful opinions, and then to talk about the same person providing false opinions. Videotape recording can be used to study and compare the verbalizations and behavior of subjects during these two situations. Other subjects (who do not know which statements are true) can then view the videotapes and be asked to evaluate the truthfulness or deceit of each statement. These judgments can be made using only visual clues (sound off), audio clues (picture off), or with both visual and audio clues.

A variety of observations of behaviors that occur more frequently during lying are summarized below. It cannot be overemphasized, however, that although these observations may be of statistical significance, they do not, in and of themselves, prove the presence or absence of lying. They accompany deception more frequently than would be expected by chance but may be present in some subjects who are not being deceitful.

Verbalization and Vocalization

The voice can send a number of messages. The words themselves can be separated from other parts of a vocal message and analyzed from a written transcript of vocalizations. A person's language, when it is deceitful, is more likely to include negative statements, irrelevant information, overgeneralized statements, fewer words in response to questions, and less personally relevant information. Statements are also more likely to appear overrehearsed and lacking in spontaneity. There may be an increased number of speech errors, including grammatical errors and slips of the tongue (B. M. DePaulo et al. 1985a; Zuckerman and Driver 1984).

Speech can also be evaluated in terms of the modulation of cadence and rate, the pitch, and response time to questions. People making deceptive statements are significantly more likely to have speech hesitations and changes in pitch (B. M. DePaulo et al. 1985a; Zuckerman and Driver 1984). They are also more likely to speak slowly and take a longer time to respond to questions, probably reflecting a need to plan their answers rather than be spontaneous. Deceptive answers to questions in an interview situation are typically more hesitant and longer in length (Harrison et al. 1978). Deceit clearly seems to place greater intellectual demands on a person than does honesty (Elliott 1979), reducing spontaneity and resulting in speech patterns that reflect a greater need to monitor what is said.

Facial Expressions and Physiological Reactions

The stereotype of a liar portrays a person who avoids eye contact, makes awkward postural changes, and smiles a lot to cover the deceit. In fact, these commonly presumed nonverbal evidences for lying are not significantly more common than would be expected by chance; perhaps this is because liars are aware of such behaviors and have relatively little difficulty in suppressing them (Ekman 1988). Nonverbal behaviors that are significantly more frequent with lying include blinking and an increased number of what have been termed *adapters*. These are nervous habits such as scratching or twiddling one's hair.

Pupil dilation is also much more common than would be expected by chance (Zuckerman and Driver 1984). The pupils are governed by the autonomic nervous system and thus are out of the liar's control. Dilation of the pupils can be a physiological sign of fear or anxiety. Other physiological signs that may indicate increased emotional arousal include flushing (blushing) or blanching of the skin, increased sweating, and changes in respiration such as hyperventilation. Breath holding or sighing are other respiratory changes that are largely under conscious control.

Smiling is an aspect of facial expression that is of great interest, one that has been extensively investigated by Ekman and colleagues (Ekman and Friesen 1982; Ekman et al. 1988). Ekman (1988) has identified and labeled different smiles. The simple (*felt*) smile reflects genuine positive emotion and is produced by the zygomatic major muscle, which pulls the lip corners up. A strong contraction of this muscle stretches the lips, pulls the checks upward, bags the skin below the eyes, and produces crows's feet wrinkles ("smile lines") beyond the eye corners.

In contrast to the felt smile, the *false smile* is intended to mislead another person into thinking a positive emotion is being experienced when it is not. Ekman describes false smiles as more asymmetrical than felt smiles, not accompanied by involvement of muscles around the eyes or inappropriate offset times, and as masks that only cover the movement of the lower face but not the reliable (more "honest") muscles of the forehead.

Ekman also describes other smiles and their muscular activation that he terms *fear smiles, contempt smiles, dampened smiles, miserable smiles* (grin and bear it), and the *Chaplin smile*. Each of these smiles represents some attempt for the smiler to mislead another person about the true underlying emotional state.

Ekman and colleagues (1988) studied smiles by using a traditional experimental design. Student nurses were videotaped while they watched a pleasant film and were asked to describe their feelings. They then watched an unpleasant film but were asked to appear as if they were watching a pleasant film. The investigators were able to identify many more false smiles in the deceptive account of the film, including some that leaked disgust or contempt. Ekman stated, however, that despite the strength of these findings, most people do not seem to use these clues when judging others. In fact, when participants who served as judges watched these tapes and were asked to determine when the nurses were smiling falsely, they could not do so any better than at a chance level (Ekman and Friesen 1974).

Body Movements

Illustrators (Ekman and Friesen 1972) are movements that are closely tied to speech, often serving to illustrate what is said. Some people automatically and actively use their hands while talking ("talk with their hands"). These movements are significantly re-duced when people are focused on exactly what it is that they are saying and when they are less spontaneous and more deliberate. A decrease in the frequency of illustrators might mean that the person is being deceptive and focused on the monitoring of the verbal content of the lie.

Although a decrease in hand movements is typically associated with deceitful statements, Bond and colleagues (1992) found that people are more likely to associate unusual movements with deceit. These authors postulated that any deviation from stereo-typed appearance or behavior is interpreted as possible evidence of deceit.

Emblems are body movements, facial expressions, or postures that have a precise meaning within a cultural group (H. G. Johnson et al. 1975). They may have a different meaning, or no meaning at all, to members of different cultures. Some examples of emblems are "giving the finger," shrugging, head nods (yes), head shakes (no), and raising an eyebrow to indicate a question of credibility. Emblems are distinctive means of nonverbal communication and, although generally under conscious control, may occur somewhat automatically, outside a person's awareness. When an emblem is in contrast to the spoken word, it suggests that the speaker is nonverbally betraying a lie. For example, a subtle head nod (yes) may be a clue that the answer "no" is a lie.

Ekman (1981) stated that no body movement, facial expression, or voice change is an indisputable sign of deceit. Rather, these signs may suggest that the speaker is uncomfortable about some aspect of the communication; intent to deceive is only one possible reason for such discomfort.

Of note, Kraut (1978) found that the same behavior—taking a long time to respond to a question—increased suspiciousness in hearers who had some reason to suspect deception but, in contrast, increased trust in the answer if the listeners had some reason to believe the answer. Kraut, like Ekman, also suggested that it is unlikely that any single behavior is invariably a signal of deception and that nonverbal behavior must be interpreted within context. The same behavior, depending on the observer's expectation, can signal deception or honesty.

Developmental Issues in the Detection of Deceit

Children develop from a position of gullibility to a more sophisticated stance, one from which it is possible to make informed decisions about the ambivalent data they receive. B. M. DePaulo and
Jordan (1982) noted that we educate our children about the real
world while simultaneously telling them stories about bears and
pigs that talk, wolves that dress up like grandmothers, black-clad
women who travel by broomstick, and a fat man dressed in red who,
once a year, flies through the air drawn by a fleet of deer. Further
adding to children's confusion about ambivalent data is the fact
that the same words said in a different manner (e.g., a statement of
praise delivered sarcastically) may connote an opposite meaning.

Just as children must be taught how to lie and must be socialized
into effective deception (see Chapter 4), they must also learn how
to read signals to decode the various forms of deception that characterize day-to-day life. When and how does this process occur?
Children tend to defer to the influence of an adult, often unquestioningly accepting what is said or suggested as fact (Ackerman
1983). This characteristic has created an enormous contemporary
problem because children may—under the "guidance" or direction
of authority figures (counselors, sexual abuse "experts")— falsely report sexual abuse (see Chapter 9). The process of becoming more
discriminating of provided information appears to be gradual
throughout childhood and is not a well-defined developmental
milestone.

Research has demonstrated that relatively small children can
identify emotions in other persons accurately and make a reasonable
assessment of the sincerity of those emotions. R. S. Feldman and
colleagues (1978) evaluated third graders who observed students
praising other students whom they were tutoring. Two situations
were presented; in one, the students were doing well and being
praised, and in the other, the students were doing poorly but were
also being praised. The third graders were able to detect some differences between the honest and dishonest communications. However, perceptiveness in differences of affective content (the genuine
emotional component) should not be interpreted as the capacity to

detect deliberate deceptiveness. A stronger conclusion is that children at this level have some ability to interpret both verbal and nonverbal communications.

In the experiment described in Chapter 4, R. S. Feldman and colleagues (1979) asked children between ages 5 and 13 years to taste either a good-tasting or bad-tasting drink and to pretend to either like or dislike both. Other children were asked to rate the videotapes of the facial expressions of the children who were the tasters and to indicate whether the taster was being truthful or deceptive. Although the children's ability to detect the false affect increased somewhat with age, this increasing ability was not very significant and basically remained at a chance level; they were wrong about as often as they were right. Of interest, however, those children who were skilled at role-taking (e.g., able to put themselves into the deceiver's shoes and imagine what the deceiver might do in the situation) were significantly better at detecting deception.

B. M. DePaulo and colleagues (1982a), noting previous research that indicated that younger children seemed to have little ability to detect deception, studied somewhat older children and adolescents. The investigators designed an experiment in which subjects between ages 11 and 18 years were exposed to an audio or audiovisual situation. They saw and/or listened to adult speakers, each of whom described six people. In addition to truthful descriptions of people they liked, disliked, were ambivalent about, or were indifferent to, the speakers also told two different kinds of lies. In one, they described someone they disliked in positive terms; in the other, they pretended to dislike someone whom they actually liked. The subjects were told about the six different types of descriptions they would receive and were asked to rate the speakers' true feelings.

The findings of this investigation were very interesting. It was consistent with the prior work of R. S. Feldman and colleagues that subjects at all age levels were able to make some discrimination of the sincerity of messages in terms of how much the senders genuinely liked an individual. Among the youngest subjects, the sincerity of liking was the only dimension in which they could differentiate truth from deception. They tended to take communications at face value, rating the senders as feeling liking whenever they were saying positive things. Furthermore, younger subjects were more likely to associate negative statements with deception, regardless of whether the messages were truthful. In other words, the younger children tended to look at the world through "rose-colored glasses"; from this perceptive, positive statements (liking) have more validity than negative statements (disliking).

By the twelfth grade, subjects were able to discriminate deceit when there was a false presentation of liking. In fact, the older subjects demonstrated a more cynical bias (as opposed to the positive bias of younger subjects) and were more likely to rate overt positive messages as lies!

B. M. DePaulo and her colleagues interpreted these findings in light of the increased life experiences accumulated by older adolescents, in contrast to the sheltered life provided to younger children. Young children are protected from harsh realities of life and are frequently told a variety of lies to spare their feelings. For example, they may be excessively praised for minor accomplishments and shielded from the painful realities of issues such as financial worries, disease, and death. Older adolescents have increased worldly experience and may, in reaction to their more naive and sheltered childhoods, become even more suspicious and cynical than the situation warrants.

How do children learn to become lie detectors? Rotenberg and colleagues (1989) addressed this in their work. They hypothesized that deception-detecting abilities depend on the capacity to determine whether the sender's nonverbal communications are consistent with the words being spoken. That is, at some point during childhood, a child develops the ability not only to understand words and read nonverbal behavior but also to correlate these two channels of communication and determine any discrepancies. In an attempt to verify this theory, the investigators, using a simple research design, videotaped presented statements that were positive, neutral, or negative in combination with different emotions, again positive, neutral, or negative. Thus, there were nine possible combinations of statements and emotions (e.g., "I like that shirt," said with a sad expression—a positive statement combined with a negative emotion). Children between ages 5 and 9 years had no difficulty identifying the emotions. They were then asked to determine whether the actor was "lying" or "truthful" in different combinations of statements and emotions. Their judgments showed that in younger kindergarten children, positive emotions (a happy face) were associated with ratings of truthfulness. However, despite the continuation of some element of this bias toward equating truthfulness with positive emotions, by the fourth grade, children were able to detect inconsistencies of emotions and words and to use this inconsistency to infer lying.

Another factor that influences a child's perception of whether someone is believable is the bias of small children toward believing adults and taking their statements at face value. Ackerman's research (1983) demonstrated that children can often accurately assess the reality of misinformation when presented by another child but will tend to believe misinformation when spoken by an adult. This bias disappears with greater maturity.

Blanck and Rosenthal (1982), using research techniques that evaluated many channels of nonverbal communication, found that as children grow older, they use both voice and body cues to decode a sender's true intentions. Interestingly, however, as female children grow older, they tend not to use the information they gather to question the veracity of the person sending a message.

Sex Differences in Lie Detection

As children mature, one necessary skill is to become a better human lie detector. Researchers are questioning whether differences may exist between the lie-detecting skills of men and women. B. M. DePaulo and colleagues (1993) recently reviewed this issue and came to some interesting conclusions.

It appears clear that women are superior to men in their ability to read nonverbal clues (B. M. DePaulo et al. 1993). They are, however, more adept at reading those cues that are easiest to regulate (facial expressions) and tend not to detect covert cues, such as body movements or very brief facial expressions (Rosenthal and DePaulo 1979). Women are more perceptive than men about how people who are telling the truth are feeling, but they are not any better, and may be worse, at detecting feelings when people are lying.

If we assume (based on the ample evidence) that the ability to read nonverbal behavior is the primary skill of human lie detection, why should a person with greater skill be poorer at the task? B. M. DePaulo et al. (1993) had an interesting and cogent answer to this paradox. They proposed that women have been socialized to become accommodating. Thus, they tend to read and accept what a person is *trying* to communicate rather than what he or she is *actually* communicating. The need to please another person takes precedence over accuracy. Women view other persons' expressions of liking or fondness (positive emotions) as more sincere than do men. But when a negative message is being conveyed, women are also more likely to accept it (accommodation) if that is how they perceive the wishes of another person.

Not all women demonstrate the accommodating pattern. Those who are more shrewd, more sophisticated, and more successful at persuading others by indirect means are less likely to be accommodating. Women who demonstrate the accommodating pattern are uncomfortable with hostility and are more likely to "just be themselves" across different situations rather than to alter their behavior from situation to situation.

A lack of skills in lie detection may have a reward. Women who are the most accommodating in the ways that they read the nonverbal cues of others are the most successful in their social lives; being too insightful about how others feel may be an interpersonal or social liability (B. M. DePaulo 1981; Rosenthal and DePaulo 1979).

B. M. DePaulo et al. (1993) concluded that women tell just as many lies as do men but that women's lies seem to support other people. With a less compassionate interpretation, women seem to achieve some of their supportiveness through deceit; men are less supportive in those ways but also more truthful.

Effects of Liar Motivation and Attractiveness on Lie Detection

One might presume that it would be more difficult to detect deception when the liar has greater motivation to deceive. However, the work of B. M. DePaulo and colleagues (B. M. DePaulo and Kirkendol 1989; B. M. DePaulo et al. 1983, 1985b, 1987, 1988) contradicts this apparently logical assumption; they found that deceit was actually easier to detect when subjects had greater motivation to lie. They hypothesized that when the subjects must increase attention to verbal content of their messages, they pay less attention to nonverbal communication channels. As a result, although the verbal message may have been convincing, the nonverbal cues (e.g., body shifts, increased voice pitch) made it easier to detect the lies of these persons.

B. M. DePaulo and her colleagues also investigated the effect of the physical attractiveness of both the originator and the target of lies. They found that deceptive messages were easier to detect when the target was believed to be an attractive person of the opposite sex. These messages were perceived as less sincere than messages directed toward persons who were believed to be less attractive. Ingratiating lies were more easily detected than noningratiating lies, especially when told to persons perceived as attractive. In later research, B. M. DePaulo and colleagues (1988) confirmed their earlier results and also found that women were more likely to show the motivational effect than men and that more attractive people were less likely to be impaired by motivation.

Sigall and Michela (1976) also investigated the role of physical attractiveness in regard to perceived messages, finding that attractiveness and self-esteem were not correlated. These authors found that attractive female subjects were more likely to believe that praise was more sincere if the sender had not seen them. Conversely, unattractive women were much more likely to believe that praise was more sincere if they had been seen.

Motivation actually appears to be an impairment to successful lying (particularly in an ingratiating manner) to attractive targets in everyday life. There are people who, with motivation and experience, appear to be quite successful liars. P. J. DePaulo and B. M. DePaulo (1989) videotaped the sales pitches of a number of salespersons. Some of these messages were for products liked by the salespersons; others were for disliked products they had to try to sell. People who watched these tapes were unable, at a level beyond chance, to determine when the salesperson was being deceptive.

B. M. DePaulo and Kirkendol (1989) concluded that some people are better liars under pressure than others. Factors that increase skill are confidence, experience at lying (e.g., sales work), comfort in the limelight, and physical attractiveness.

Interviewer Influences on Lying Behavior

Interviewing style can influence the veracity of an interviewee's statements. Stiff and Miller (1986) found that giving positive feedback to a person who is making false statements will increase deceitfulness. Apparently the liar, who is "reading" the target, is inclined to increase the behavior that is being reinforced. In contrast, a person who is making truthful statements when receiving negative feedback is likely to become even more truthful in an effort to establish veracity.

This technique has practical application in the case of a person suspected of pseudologia fantastica. I have found that instead of questioning the veracity of a pseudologue's statements, it is much more diagnostically useful to indicate considerable interest in what is being said. So encouraged, the pseudologue progressively escalates the stories until it is clear that the productions are false.

Learning to Be a Better Lie Detector

There is solid evidence that when people lie, they often provide detection clues through discrepant verbal and nonverbal messages. Logic dictates that people can learn to recognize and interpret these discrepant messages in order to become increasingly better lie detectors. To some degree, this process comes with maturity. There is also evidence that some people may be inherently better lie detectors than others. The evidence that most people can be taught to become better liars is not, however, very compelling.

Most research studies have suggested that most people can detect deceit at a rate slightly greater than chance (B. M. DePaulo et al. 1980). A few individuals may have more exceptional abilities to detect lying, and their successful detection rate may reach 80% or 90% (Ekman and O'Sullivan 1991). Why most people are not more successful at detecting lies is, of itself, an interesting question. Perhaps, as suggested by B. M. DePaulo (1981), many people unconsciously view lie detection as a liability rather than a skill.

It stands to reason that if people do leak detection clues when lying and if some people are skilled in identifying such clues, then it should be possible to teach these clues to train people to be better lie detectors. Such efforts have met with mixed results at best. Zuckerman and colleagues (1984, 1985) showed videotapes of people lying and people telling the truth to subjects, asking them to determine whether the messages were truthful or deceptive. Some videotapes displayed both speech and face, others face only, and still others speech only. Subjects were given feedback about the accuracy of their judgments. Modest improvements in lie detection occurred but only in the speech-only and face-plus-speech videotapes. Increased accuracy occurred when the subjects evaluated a specific sender, but the skill did not generalize to other deceivers. In other words, with experience, one can learn to detect deceit in an individual about whom one has increasing information, but this ability does not extend to other people.

Kohnken (1987) studied four groups of experienced police officers who watched and heard videotaped statements, both true and false. One group of officers was told to attend to the senders' facial nonverbal behavior, another was to pay attention to paralinguistic behavior (e.g., vocal pitch), another group was instructed to pay attention to the content of the statements, and the last group was provided with no specific instructions. Each group (except the last) received a 45-minute training session on the specific clues for which they were to look. The police officers in this study were not able to learn to detect deception at a rate greater than that expected by chance. Those who paid attention only to the words were incorrect more frequently than would be expected by chance. Of note, it was not demonstrated that the length of their police work experience made a difference in their abilities to discern true statements from false. Furthermore, there was an inverse correlation with the subjects' confidence in their judgments; the more certain they were that they were right, the more likely they were to be wrong!

Two German researchers (Fiedler and Walka 1993) have been more successful in training people to be better at detecting deceit. From their review of research on nonverbal detection cues, Fiedler and Walka picked the seven cues from the Zuckerman and Driver's meta-analysis (1984) that appeared to have the greatest diagnostic validity:

1. Disguised smiling
2. Lack of head movement
3. Increased rate of self-adapters (e.g., movements such as scratching one's head)
4. Increased pitch of voice
5. Reduced rate of speech
6. Pause fillers ("uh ," "er")
7. Less harmonic and congruent nonverbal behavior from the various communication channels

These investigators used a somewhat different topic from the usual paradigm (whether a speaker likes or dislikes another person) to differentiate truth and deceit. Instead, in an interview situation, they had the senders talk about whether they had been involved in common petty crimes, such as riding on a public bus without a ticket, minor theft (e.g., of newspapers), and so forth. In these videotaped interviews, the senders were truthful half the time and lied half the time.

Subjects, whose task was to judge the credibility of statements, were divided into three groups. A control group received no training but used whatever general knowledge about lie detection they had acquired in their life experiences; the second group received information about the seven nonverbal diagnostic cues; and the third group received not only the information about nonverbal cues but also feedback information about the accuracy of their judgments for the first 16 trials.

The results of this experiment were very interesting. All subjects performed more accurately than the chance level in determining the veracity of statements. The group taught about specific nonverbal cues performed better than the uninformed control group in determining when a statement was false but did not gain much expertise from either feedback or greater experience (number of trials). In determining the veracity of "true" statements, all subjects were more accurate with increasing experience, particularly those with training and feedback. It is interesting that feedback did not seem to improve accuracy as much as might have been anticipated. This finding is consistent with some previous research (Brandt et al. 1980) that suggests that increasing the number of trials (increasing familiarity) initially increases the accuracy of truth–deception judgments, but the accuracy rate then declines. Brandt and colleagues suggested that as the observers' familiarity with the sender increases, the observers may become burdened with information, which results in a decreased efficiency in the accuracy of their judgments. This explanation may be one reason that one spouse often has difficulty in determining when the other is lying!

The above brief review of whether persons can learn to become better lie detectors suggests that a significant improvement in the skill of detecting deception is not probable for most people. However, a few persons may have an inherent talent for such an ability. Let us now turn our attention to those people who presumably are "professional" lie detectors and look at their abilities for recognizing deceit.

Professional Human Lie Detectors

The movie *Maverick* shows the exploits of a fanciful master poker player, Bret Maverick. The protagonist wins at poker, easily defeating his fellow gamblers, including the glamorous Ms. Annabelle Bradford. At one point, he charitably lets her know that she had tipped herself by nervously tapping her teeth. In the climactic big game, she is again defeated while attempting to bluff with a poor hand. She angrily asked Maverick how he knew. "Breath holding," he replies with a double entendre, "You hold your breath when you get excited."

To what extent can a person develop skills to detect deception? Are there professionals who have mastered the art of reading the nonverbal communications of others? Information presented in the preceding section suggests that most people are not particularly adept at detecting lies, and they do not seem to improve their skill with training. Can someone such as Bret Maverick really "read" the telltale signs of other poker players, or is it merely the stuff that makes good movies? One scientist, David Hayano (1980, 1988) of California State University at Northridge, studied this question and has come to some interesting conclusions. He noted that "our understanding of what professional poker players do over the cardroom table may very well be significant in detecting deception and distorted structures of communication in everyday life" (p. 119).

Dr. Hayano describes three levels of poker players. Beginners and amateurs have no ability to control their bodies and are highly prone to leaking information. They readily and unambiguously reveal the strength of their cards through "tells." More experienced players can control their bodies and can sometimes successfully bluff others. It is the skills of the most experienced professional poker players that are so fascinating. They possess a "startling accuracy" in their ability to gauge the exact hand values of opposing players. They literally "read" amateurs. To develop and use these skills of decoding messages, the professional may keep long—memorized and possibly written—lists of the playing styles and idiosyncrasies of hundreds of regular opponents. They also know that staring at an opponent may increase the other's anxiety and thus result in greater leakage of information.

Strategies to put other professional players off guard may include efforts to neutralize all of one's own nonverbal communications, the proverbial "poker face." They may go so far as to wear dark glasses in order to hide as much of the face as possible and to obscure any possible detection of pupillary dilation that can occur with excitement and autonomic arousal. A second strategy is to keep up such a barrage of behaviors, verbal and nonverbal, that it is difficult to separate out the real messages, which are lost in the noise; these players continuously talk and gesticulate. Yet another strategy to camouflage one's potential "tells" is to make unpredictable shifts of mood and changes from silence to constant talking and back to silence. All of these strategies are attempts to hide the inadvertent leakage of nonverbal messages. Further complicating the detection of deceit among poker players, some players use "false tells" and "antitells." In the former situation, a player may go to elaborate lengths to create the appearance of a tell; for example, coughing when bluffing. The false tell may be consciously used to deceive with very large pots. Antitells are movements that appear to be tells but are displayed in a random manner to confuse opponents.

Hayano concluded that even among the professionals, most are more competent at sending false information than they are at accurately decoding information. The ability to decode is attained only by keeping exhaustive mental or written notes or by personal familiarity. In this respect, the considerable skills of professional poker players reflect the deception and detection abilities in everyday life.

I now address another group of professional lie detectors—those officials who must judge the honesty of others on a day-to-day basis. Two groups of these officials—law enforcement officers and customs inspectors—have been studied for their skills in detecting deceit in others.

Customs inspectors must make numerous rapid decisions about whom they will challenge, and possibly search, out of the many people who enter the United States. In an experimental setting, a group of experienced customs inspectors was compared with a group of laypersons by using the technique of videotaped mock inspection interviews (Kraut and Poe 1980). The videotapes were of a variety of airplane passenger volunteers, half of whom had been given contraband goods. The volunteers were offered a cash prize if they were successful in fooling the inspectors. Travelers who were given contraband proved to be good liars, and both laypersons and customs inspectors were less suspicious of them than of the travelers not carrying contraband. Of importance was the finding that laypersons were better at determining who was a smuggler than were the customs inspectors!

Despite the knowledge that they were participating in an experimental task, the customs inspectors could not let go of firmly held prejudices that certain characteristics (e.g., age, sex, race, and social class) are associated with smuggling. Characteristics used by both laypersons and customs inspectors to initiate a request for a search included behaviors such as short answers, body shifts, poor eye contact, volunteering of extra information, evasion of direct answers, and general nervousness. This experiment strongly suggested that members of this group of professional lie detectors were no better than laypersons at their task, and that they had, in fact, developed stereotypical beliefs (inaccurate) about whom to search.

B. M. DePaulo and Pfeifer (1986) evaluated the skill of law enforcement officers to detect deception. They administered a standardized detection test to three samples of more than 100 subjects each. The test consisted of judging the truthfulness of audiotape messages (half of which were deceitful). The three experimental groups of subjects included undergraduate students who had no special experience at detecting deceit, new recruits to a federal law enforcement training program who had some limited on-the-job experience at detecting deceit, and a group of highly experienced law enforcement officers working at jobs in which the detection of deceit is very important.

In this experiment, the accuracy rate of all the subjects was barely statistically significant at 53.6%. Furthermore, there were no differences among the three groups. Students did as well as the law enforcement officers, and inexperienced officers did as well as more experienced ones. All subjects felt confident in the accuracy of their judgments even though they were wrong almost half of the time. The most experienced officers demonstrated a negative correlation between accuracy and confidence. In other words, the more certain they were that they were right, the more likely they were to be wrong.

The above studies involving law enforcement officers might be criticized because the settings were artificial, that is, not in the usual line of police work. Aldert Vrij (1993) dealt with this issue by conducting a carefully designed experimental study in which an actor dressed as a police officer interrogated other actors who were being questioned about whether they had a set of earphones in their pockets. These actors denied possession at all times, although half of them did have earphones (thus, 50% of their statements were truthful). Twenty standardized interrogations were videotaped (10 truthful and 10 deceitful) and put together into one tape (with a 15-second pause for the subjects to indicate their judgment of truth or deception, as well as their degree of confidence in their decision).

Each of 92 Dutch detectives, with an average experience of 17 years on the police force, viewed the tape. The results of this investigation indicated that although the detectives were confident in their decisions (and as a group tended to rate the same interrogations as truthful or lying), they were accurate only 49% of the time. Once again, consistent with the other studies detailed above, there was a trend (not statistically significant) for confidence to be inversely related to accuracy. The detectives (incorrectly) used clothing (e.g., dirty clothing equals criminal attitude), degree of smiling, and degree of hand or arm movements to make their determinations of deceit. The detectives used the last criterion despite the fact that deceit has been shown in previous research to be associated with fewer hand or arm movements. The conclusion from this study is that experience may cause overconfidence in one's abilities and may lead to the use of stereotyped criteria for judgments, thereby detracting a person from learning and using more effective cues.

A large-scale study of persons of several different occupations confirmed data from the studies described above, while revealing one startling difference. Ekman and O'Sullivan (1991) found that only members of the United States Secret Service could significantly differentiate truth from deceit by using a standardized videotape test. (The videotapes consisted of nursing students describing their feelings as pleasant while watching a film, whether or not the film was pleasant or gruesome.) Persons from other occupations, including robbery investigators, federal polygraphers, judges, psychiatrists, and college students, performed at a chance level.

However, among all groups, and especially among the Secret Service agents, some individuals were especially good lie detectors and were correct 80% or more of the time. Twenty-nine percent of the Secret Service agents reached that level of accuracy; among psychiatrists (the second-place group), only 12% were at least 80% accurate. Persons who demonstrated a high level of accuracy were more likely to attend to nonverbal cues alone and to nonverbal clues in relation to speech. Those persons who demonstrated a low level of lie detection attended only to speech. Another skill of the highly accurate subjects was their ability to detect microexpressions of emotions (very brief emotional lapses that are out of place).

The authors speculated that perhaps one reason that Secret Service agents were superior in detecting deceit is that their job often involves scanning for suspicious persons in large crowds. In addition, their work in interrogating people has led them to believe that most people are telling the truth. This is in contrast to other law enforcement officers who believe that everybody lies to them.

The Ekman–O'Sullivan study confirmed previous work in finding that most groups, including law enforcement officers, have no special skills in detecting deceit. Furthermore, their data demonstrated no relation between a person's confidence in lie-detecting ability and accuracy at the task.

Professor Ray Bull (1989) of Glasgow, Scotland, called attention to a number of police recruitment advertisements and police training books that imply that detecting deception is simple. These advertisements suggest that training to detect behavioral and speech clues can increase one's abilities. With the exception of two unpublished studies (which could not be critically analyzed as to their validity), Bull found no evidence that training enhances a police officer's ability to detect deception. He concluded that the advertisements and training books were themselves deceptive.

In summary, it is apparent that, with two exceptions—professional poker players and Secret Service agents—persons whose jobs should involve a high degree of skill in detecting lies have no more skill at this function than do laypersons. Unfortunately, however, these persons often deceive themselves by having false confidence in their abilities. They use the wrong cues, often based on stereotyped prejudices, to make their decisions.

Summary

The detection of deceit is an everyday skill practiced by everyone. The primary means by which false statements are separated from true statements are by verbal messages that are inconsistent with other facts known to the listener and by inconsistency between the verbal message and nonverbal behavior. Detecting deceit is a developmental skill; children progressively learn how to read nonverbal messages and how to compare these with the verbal message. With more life experiences, they also learn to evaluate spoken words more critically. Most people, from children through adults, have a bias toward assuming that what is said is the truth. This bias helps facilitate social interaction; being too cynical is a social liability.

Most people can detect deceit at a rate that is greater than by chance but not by much. Many people whose jobs should be associated with greater lie-detecting skill, such as police, are confident in their abilities to detect lying, but they are self-deceptive; their ability to detect deception is no better than that of the general population. A small group of people have exceptional skills in detecting deceit in others. From either specific training or innate abilities, they are attuned to nonverbal communications and to the leakage of microexpressions of affect.

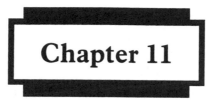

Chapter 11

Technological Detection of Deceit

Personally, I have grave reservations about so-called lie detector tests.

—Secretary of State George Shultz,
December 20, 1985

Faced with the importance of knowing when someone is lying and recognizing the fallibility of humans as lie detectors, people have, through the ages, sought external means to determine the presence of deceit. In recent years, the polygraph has been used for that purpose. The extensive use of this device to monitor the honesty of employees, governmental officials, and criminals (among others) has been notably controversial.

Brief History of Lie Detection

Efforts to detect deception undoubtedly extend back to the first interactions among humans. One of the first recorded incidents is in the biblical story of two women who each claimed a baby as her own. They appeared before King Solomon, who, to resolve the conflict, offered to cut the infant in half and divide it between them. The true mother was distraught, and the false mother agreed with the decision; thus, Solomon awarded the infant to the former. Although this story can be interpreted at several different levels, Kleinmuntz and Szucko (1984a) pointed out that Solomon made his decision on the basis of the emotional arousal of the truthful mother. This is in contrast to modern lie detection, which generally assumes that emotional arousal is associated with deceit. Kleinmuntz and Szucko questioned whether King Solomon's decision would have been the same if he had relied on a late-twentieth-century polygrapher!

Through the years, and in widely differing cultures, a variety of different methods have been used to detect lies (Trovillo 1939, 1940). These methods have often consisted of an "ordeal," the successful completion of which was interpreted as truthfulness or honesty. Among these ordeals was the red-hot iron method of the Bedouin of Arabia: conflicting witnesses were required to lick a hot iron rod, and the one whose tongue was burned was considered to be the liar. In India, accused persons were required to chew dry rice and then spit it out; if it remained dry or if blood tinged it, the accused person was considered guilty. A similar technique was used during the Spanish Inquisition. The accused person was required to swallow a piece of bread and cheese; if it stuck in the suspect's palate or throat, the person was judged guilty. Each of the above situations was based on the assumption that decreased saliva flow (which we now know to be associated with anxiety and sympathetic autonomic nervous system arousal) pointed to deception. Although a guilty person might experience *more* anxiety, Trovillo pointed out that an innocent person might also experience anxiety because of the fear of not being believed or because of the prospect of having to lick a red-hot iron.

According to one story, in the Middle Ages, a nobleman who was suspicious of his wife's fidelity sought the assistance of his adviser. The adviser sat next to the wife during dinner, laid his hand on her wrist, and conversed with her. At one point when he deliberately mentioned the name of the suspected paramour, the woman's pulse quickened, but no such response was noted at the mention of her husband's name. Allegedly, a confession was subsequently elicited from her (reported in Trovillo 1939).

These "low-tech" lie-detection techniques were supplanted by technological advances during the early part of the twentieth century. The work of psychophysiologists, who investigated the physiological changes associated with emotions, was put to use by the Italian criminologist Lombros. He and his colleague Mosso used changes in pulse rate and in the blood volume of a person's limbs to interpret the truthfulness of answers given by suspected criminals during interrogations. Later, Benussi (another Italian) related lying to changes in respiration, and Marston (a Harvard student) reported correlations between lying and systolic blood pressure. One of the first polygraphs was constructed by Larson, a Berkeley medical student working with the police department. This device measured blood pressure, pulse rate, and respiration. Later, Larson and Keeler constructed the prototype of the modern polygraph, one small enough to fit into a compact box the size of a small suitcase. A measure of the galvanic skin response (the degree of electroconductivity determined by perspiration) was later added to the physiological parameters already measured.

Improvements in technology have increased the quality of such measurements and have led to smaller equipment, but the modern polygraph continues to measure the same physiological parameters as in the 1930s—pulse and relative blood pressure, depth and rate of respiration, and skin conductivity.

Modern Technological Lie Detection

Technological lie detection is based on the assumption that physiological responses to anxiety or guilt caused by untruthful statements can be objectively measured. Thus, several different psychophysiological responses are commonly evaluated in a polygraph interview. Before reviewing the various techniques used by polygraph operators and the criticisms associated with these techniques, I first consider several actual cases in which polygraphs were used.

Roger Keith Coleman was convicted of the brutal murder and rape of his sister-in-law. He steadfastly insisted that he was innocent, and two national news magazines (*Time* and *Newsweek*) published major stories that detailed the weakness of the case against him (e.g., after his conviction, four persons had come forward to state that they had heard someone else confess to the crime) (J. Johnson 1992; Kaplan 1992). Unfortunately for Coleman, his situation was prejudiced by a prior conviction for attempted rape. In a last-ditch attempt to prove his innocence and save his life, Coleman asked for a polygraph examination. This request was granted by Douglas Wilder, then Governor of Virginia. The polygraph test was administered 12 hours before the scheduled execution. It was publicly announced that Coleman had failed the polygraph test, and he was put to death in the Virginia electric chair later that night (*Washington Post*, May 11, 1992). For its article on the execution, the *Washington Post* interviewed Professor David Lykken, a leading critic of polygraphs. He was quoted as saying, "I was horrified to hear about that polygraph test. A polygraph test can't measure lying. It measures arousal. How anyone on the brink of execution could pass a polygraph is beyond me."

Was Governor Wilder a modern-day Pontius Pilate providing bloodthirsty "law-and-order" voters with their wish for vengeance? Was he merely misguided and uninformed, making the best decision possible for a layperson? Or does the polygraph really measure that which its proponents claim?

Kleinmuntz and Szucko (1984b) recounted the case of a police officer accused of burglary. The officer had reported the burglary in a timely manner, but because of suspicious circumstances, he was charged with the crime. An offer was made to drop the charges if he submitted to a polygraph examination. Because he feared that he would be judged guilty if he refused, the officer reluctantly agreed; he failed the test.

During the investigation, it was learned that the officer had violated regulations by agreeing to watch the house in question during his off-duty hours. He feared reprisals for breaking regulations with his moonlighting activities, and he feared the prospect of going to prison for conviction of a felony. Caught in the bind of not wanting to confess to the more minor infraction, he had reacted with progressively increased anxiety to each of the questions posed to him. Fortunately, expert testimony convinced the police commissioners that there is no unique physiological response to deception and that false-positive rates (innocent persons judged to be deceptive) are in the range of 30%–50%.

Lykken (1974) has collected similar case histories, including that of a man who failed his polygraph test (but was innocent) and was imprisoned for murder.

The popular CBS television show *60 Minutes* dramatized problems with the polygraph examination in a program aired in 1986 (Saxe 1991). The *60 Minutes* crew used the CBS-owned magazine *Popular Photography* as a front for a mock theft. Four separate polygraphers were selected from the telephone directory and told that more than $500 worth of camera equipment had been stolen, almost definitely by an insider, and that there were four suspects. No polygrapher was told about the other polygraphers, and each polygrapher was told that a different one of the four suspects was probably the guilty party. In each situation, the polygrapher found the "fingered" party to be deceptive and strived to get that person to confess. Of course, nothing had been stolen, and each of the four polygraphers had selected a different "guilty party." Saxe noted that the demonstration was very clever but that it also involved deception; CBS employees had lied to the polygraphers. Whether the polygraphers, in turn, were lying to please their customer or were self-deceptive was not determined.

This television program was a topical dramatization of concerns about the polygraph fever (Biddle 1986; Dujack 1986; Joyce 1984) that was sweeping the United States in the mid-1980s. Polygraph tests were being increasingly used (or misused) by employers who wanted to screen potential new employees and check on established employees for possible misconduct. These examinations reportedly often went beyond their ostensible purpose and invaded the personal lives of the individuals being examined. It was estimated that during the mid-1980s as many as 1 million persons were administered a total of 2 million polygraph examinations per year.

Enthralled by the potential strength of technology to ferret out disloyal and dishonest federal employees, the Reagan administration launched a plan for extensive polygraph testing at all levels of the government. This plan was derailed by the vociferous objections of then-Secretary of State George Shultz, who announced that he had no intention of subjecting himself to such a test (Gwertzman 1985). A well-publicized document published by the U.S. Government Office of Technology Assessment (1985) cast further doubt on the effectiveness of polygraph examinations. It particularly addressed concerns about pre-employment screening in which no efficacy for the polygraph had ever been demonstrated and the use of which had the potential to adversely affect the careers of many innocent people. In 1988, despite the vigorous objections of the American Polygraph Association, some law enforcement agencies, and some major employers, Congress restricted use of the polygraph in the private sector. However, major exceptions to the restrictions were made, especially in situations dealing with national security.

Polygraph Apparatus

The polygraph used today is a compact piece of equipment about the size of an attaché case; the polygrapher can travel to wherever the examinee is located. The mechanical essentials of the polygraph include a motorized paper feeder and styluses that record (on paper) the input of transducers. These transducers measure electrodermal activity, heart rate and relative blood pressure, and respiration rate and depth. A marking device indicates when questions are asked. Except for improvements in design, the polygraph has remained essentially unchanged over the past 60 years.

The polygraph record (the paper graph with its multiple lines) is scored according to the extent of deviations from baseline that occur in response to certain questions. Systematic questioning yields numerical scores, and recent advances have included computer-generated scoring systems (Raskin et al. 1989).

Polygraph Examination

The technical aspects of measuring the standard physiological parameters are straightforward. The major areas of contention over polygraph tests are 1) the way in which the questions (the interrogation) are framed and asked and 2) the interpretation of polygraph responses to these questions and answers. Three types of interrogation have been promulgated.

Relevant Question Test

The relevant question test is the oldest and simplest method used. A series of neutral questions is asked in order to obtain a baseline and then the "relevant question" is posed. For example, "What is your name?" "Are you sitting down?" "Did you steal the money from the cash register?"

Control Question Test

The control question test is the most common technique currently used. It is based on certain questions in response to which the individual is very likely to lie. These responses, assumed to be lies, are compared with the responses to the relevant question. Thus, the polygrapher seeks to identify a person's response to lies about relatively innocuous issues and to determine whether this pattern is present when the person answers the relevant question. For example, "What is your name?" "Did you ever steal anything?" "Are you sitting down?" "Did you ever tell a lie?" "What is the color of your hair?" "Did you take the money from the cash register?" Obviously, essentially everyone has stolen something at some point in life, and everyone has lied. The person being interrogated, however, may be very fearful of admitting to any previous misdemeanors for fear of being identified as an untrustworthy person.

The importance of the interview that precedes the actual polygraph examination was highlighted when Elaad (1993) suggested that the examiner use transactional analysis techniques to enhance the physiological responses. That is, Elaad proposed that the examiner set up a parent-child interaction that reinforces childlike behavior on the part of the examinee, thus increasing the probability of inducing guilt feelings in the examinee. Even setting aside ethical concerns, it is apparent from these suggestions that this examination has a very large subjective component, even though it is supposed to be objective in nature.

Guilty Knowledge Test

The guilty knowledge test (GKT) is used less frequently by polygraphers, perhaps because they have poor understanding of its potential discriminative power. Also, the GKT requires that the polygrapher have specific knowledge of the crime, and the interrogation must be carefully constructed. The GKT presumes that the guilty person has more detailed knowledge about the crime (or other activity at issue) than does an innocent party. The interrogator poses a series of multiple-choice questions. Although anybody might have a random increased physiological response to any one question, a person who has an increased physiological response to many of the correct relevant multiple-choice questions is more likely to be guilty. Thus, a pattern can be established that permits the construction of mathematical odds of deception or truthfulness. For example, "What is your name?" "Was the money in the cash register mostly 10s, 20s, or 50s?" "Are you sitting down?" "Was the money in the cash divider or under the cash divider?" "What color is your hair?" "How much money was stolen: $50, $100, or $150?"

If the money stolen was primarily $50 bills that were under the cash divider and the amount of money was $150, and no one else had access to this information, the odds for an increased physiological response to the correct answer in each situation can be calculated. The person has a 1-in-3 chance of knowing the size of the bills, a 1-in-2 chance of knowing the place of the money, and a 1-in-3 chance of knowing the correct amount. One-third times one-half times one-third equals 1 in 18. Thus, the chance is only a little more than 5% that an innocent person would have an increased physiological response to all three of the correct answers.

In some situations, the GKT would have powerful discriminative value to determine "truth" or identity. Lykken (1991) illustrated how it would have been technically possible to have established whether John Demjanjuk was, in fact, "Ivan the Terrible" of the Treblinka concentration camp.

The sketchy descriptions of these three different interview techniques are obviously simplistic, but they outline the general principles involved. Readers who want specific details may wish to review other source material (Lykken 1974, 1991; Raskin et al. 1989).

Theoretical Bases for Polygraph Interpretation

The polygraph measures physiological responsiveness, nothing more, and as such it determines whether an individual is in a state of autonomic nervous system arousal. More specifically, it determines whether the sympathetic autonomic nervous system has been activated and whether adrenergic neurotransmitters (epinephrine and norepinephrine—also known as adrenaline and noradrenaline) have been released. Such activity occurs with anxiety, fear, and anger. No specific physiological signs of deception or guilt exist. Thus, an increased physiological response (e.g., an increased heart rate or increased electrical conduction in the skin) may mean only that the person is anxious, fearful, or angry. It requires a jump in logic to assume that the anxiety is due to guilt or fear of detection. Alternative explanations of a person's anxiety must be considered, as in the case of the police officer described above.

A person being examined is more likely to react with anxiety to questions related to deception if he or she believes that the polygraph does accurately detect lying. Some examiners make elaborate attempts to convince the person being interrogated that it is impossible to fool the machine. The polygraph then becomes an elaborate stage prop for an interview that may precipitate a confession. Therefore, both the police and the polygraph examiners may develop an increasing belief and reliance on a procedure that in and of itself has limited validity (Lykken 1974, 1987a, 1987b).

Validity and Reliability of the Polygraph

Leading scientists have raised major questions concerning both the validity and reliability of the polygraph. *Validity* is a scientific term used to evaluate whether something measures what it is supposed to measure (i.e., whether the polygraph measures deception or something else). *Reliability* is a measurement of the consistency of results when the same instrument and technique are used by different examiners, or with different examinations at different times. The *60 Minutes* program described earlier in this chapter certainly calls into question both the validity and reliability of polygraph examinations.

The degree to which polygraphers have achieved accuracy has varied widely. Szucko and Kleinmuntz (1981) used an experimental study (mock thievery) to investigate the capabilities of six polygraphers with different experience levels in their attempts to evaluate truthfulness. They found that the best interpreter incorrectly classified 18% of truthful subjects as untruthful; the worst interpreter incorrectly classified 55% of truthful subjects. It is important to note that the most experienced (8 years) polygrapher had the highest false-positive rate.

The same investigators also studied polygraphers in actual situations (Kleinmuntz and Szucko 1984a). They used 120 polygraph tracings that had been obtained in actual investigations of robbery. Fifty of these tracings represented polygraph interviews of persons who were later proven guilty because they confessed, and 50 were from persons later proven innocent because someone else confessed to the crime. Twenty tracings were indeterminate and helped to illustrate that not all examinations provide clear-cut data. Control and relevant questions had been asked during these polygraph examinations. Unfortunately, the results of these evaluations did not show any striking differences between the genuine criminals and the innocent people. The range of overall accuracy was between 63% and 76% for the six polygraphers, with a false-positive range of 18%–50%. Although there was modest reliability among the judges (i.e., the polygraphers made similar determinations), the interpreters were consistently more likely to label a suspect untruthful than truthful. The authors concluded that the control question test as currently used is flawed but that the GKT has promise for greater validity. Other investigators have also found that the rate of false-positive rates is consistently higher than that of false-negative results and that overall accuracy falls into the range of 80%–90% at best (Office of Technology Assessment 1985).

David Raskin, a professor of psychology at the University of Utah, has supported the responsible use of the polygraph and frequently disagrees with Lykken (Raskin and Kircher 1987; Raskin and Podlensky 1979). He and his colleagues believe that with skilled, well-trained examiners who are using a structured control question technique, accuracy can exceed 90% (Raskin et al. 1989). However, even Raskin has said, "There's a great disparity between the potential of the polygraph and the way it's actually used. . . . As far as I'm concerned, the whole Department of Defense polygraphy department is atrocious—and almost all the federal examiners are trained at the DOD institution. Polygraphers in law enforcement train at private schools and most of these are terrible" (Davis 1992, p. 92).

A consistent finding is that polygraphers report more false-positive results than false-negative results; that is, more truth-tellers are reported as deceptive than deceptive persons are reported as truth-telling. Kleinmuntz and Szucko (1984b) have analyzed this bias in interpretation and proposed several reasons for it. They suggest that because polygraphers are paid by employers and administrators, they are motivated to identify guilty suspects and uncover cases of deception to justify their fees. Furthermore, the tendency is to err on the side of caution. It is deemed safer to fire a trustworthy employee (because of a false-positive test result) than to risk a security breach (because of a false-negative test result). Also, polygraphers are much more likely to get feedback in the form of client complaints when an employee incorrectly classified as truthful proves to be otherwise. In contrast, the polygrapher is unlikely to hear about the honest individual who was unjustly fired or perhaps never hired. Thus, the bias is in favor of the organization rather than the person being interrogated.

The overwhelming majority of polygraphers are not scientists or statisticians. They have little understanding of the principles of validity and reliability, and they often receive no follow-up information on the accuracy of their determinations. As a result, they frequently "become victims of their own deceptive art" (Lykken 1991, p. 218). In other words, they come to self-deceptively believe that they can detect deception when, in fact, they cannot.

Yet another confounding variable in assessing deception with the polygraph test is that skilled liars may be difficult or impossible to detect. People with antisocial personality disorder (also known as sociopaths or psychopaths) may have less autonomic reactivity than people without this disorder; thus, they may show fewer physiological changes on the polygraph (Lykken 1957; Schmauk 1970). Regardless of potential differences in physiological reactivity, people with antisocial personality disorder are usually skilled liars who have little guilt about their behavior (see Chapter 6). As a consequence, polygraph detection of their lies would theoretically be more difficult.

Lykken (1974) provided some mathematical models for calculating the probability of detecting a guilty party with the polygraph examination. For example, imagine that a group of 1,000 government employees is screened to search for one spy. If the polygraph is about 80% accurate in determining who is telling the truth (20% false-positive and 10% false-negative), then 200 persons would be falsely accused, and there would still be a 10% chance that the actual spy would pass the test. In truth, because spies are trained to foil the polygraph (see below) the probability of detecting such an individual would actually be much lower. These numbers highlight the impractical aspect of the use of the polygraph to detect misbehavior that occurs at a low incidence.

Foiling the Polygraph

The only thing that the polygraph can measure is changes in physiological activity. Can a person deliberately induce physiological changes that can mask other physiological activity or provide misleading information?

> Floyd "Buzz" Fay, who was falsely convicted of murder on the basis of a failed polygraph examination, took it on himself to become a polygraph expert during his 2½ years of wrongful imprisonment. Fay coached 27 inmates, all of whom freely confessed to him that they were guilty, on how to "beat" the control question polygraph test. After only 20 minutes of instruction, 23 of the 27 (85%) were successful in foiling the polygraph examination. (Kleinmuntz and Szucko 1984b)

Techniques used by persons who are attempting to foil a polygraph examination include recognizing the control questions and using this recognition to deliberately depart from usual breathing patterns, tighten the anal sphincter, and bite one's tongue (Biddle 1986). Although many proponents of the polygraph are aware of these techniques and claim they can detect them, a recently published scientific study lends credence to the effectiveness of countermeasures to defeat the polygraph. Honts and colleagues (1994) found that after training guilty subjects to recognize control questions and to use a physical or mental countermeasure, 50% of the subjects were able to fool the polygraph examiner. Physical techniques included biting the tongue or pressing toes to the floor. The mental technique was to count backward by seven. The authors noted that these countermeasures were difficult to detect, either through observation by the examiner or on the polygraph record.

A concrete and dramatic example of foiling the polygraph is the case of Aldrich Ames. Ames—who for many years leaked information to the Soviet government and was possibly the most damaging American traitor in recent decades—foiled the polygraph twice during routine examinations in 1986 and 1991 (Safire 1994).

Recommendations for Polygraph Use

The polygraph evolved from the work of psychophysiologists, yet at present (with relatively few exceptions), it is used outside the science of psychology. Few polygraphers have much knowledge of psychology; conversely, psychologists have, on the whole, not ventured into what many of them regard to be pseudoscience. Despite this paradox, the polygraph interview is a psychological test, as are Rorschach, Thematic Apperception Test, or Memory for Designs. Each of these tests requires skill for administration, experience for interpretation, and a mature comprehensive view of both the strengths and limitations of the test; a polygraph test is no different. Thus, I propose that the polygraph examination be conducted as a psychological test that is administered only by licensed professional psychologists who meet minimal educational standards and who adhere to specified ethical principles.

Advanced Technological Assessment of Deceit

The polygraph is not the only technological instrument used to assess deceit. Efforts have been made to use electroencephalogram (EEG) responses to stimuli in order to detect deception. Lawrence Farwell, a scientist in Washington, D.C., claims that EEG responses to familiar words are different from those to unfamiliar words. Thus, in a manner similar to the GKT described earlier in this chapter, a suspect may be presented with a series of different words, some relevant and others irrelevant. If the person being interrogated consistently reacts to some words as if they were familiar but about which he or she should have no knowledge, the assumption is that the individual has some knowledge about that area of the investigation. Through this technique, Farwell was able to correctly identify 17 of 21 Federal Bureau of Investigation agents. This type of EEG lie-detector research is clearly preliminary and requires confirmation and refinement. However, even in its preliminary stages, it is controversial. Janlon Golman, director of the American Civil Liberties Union, has called it a "frightening invasion of privacy" (Witkin 1993, p. 49).

Summary

The search for a valid, reliable mechanism to measure truthfulness and deceit began long ago and continues to the present. Although the polygraph is widely used, it is fraught with conceptual confusion and misuse in its application. According to Steinbrook (1992, p. 123), "The polygraph appeals to an often simplistic desire for certainty in the face of complexity and to a misplaced faith in the power of a machine."

When an evaluation is ethically conducted by a skilled professional, the polygraph (and its inevitable technological successors) can provide important data. As with the administration of any psychological test, the results of a polygraph examination must be interpreted with a clear understanding of what it measures (emotional arousal, not deception) and the limitations of what can be concluded from the findings. It is strongly recommended that the polygraph be recognized as a psychological test and that its use be limited to trained and certified psychologists.

Chapter 12

Therapeutic Approaches for the Deceitful Person

No man can be secret, except he give himself a little scope of dissimulation; which is, as it were, but the skirts or train of secrecy.

—Sir Francis Bacon

Lying is a ubiquitous behavior and is not of itself an indication for psychiatric or psychological treatment. Relatively few persons ever seek treatment for an acknowledged problem with lying; when they do, it is usually at the instigation of another person. However, psychotherapists encounter deceit on a daily basis. Most frequently, this deceit is in the form of self-deception. The very heart of insight-oriented psychotherapy lies in the therapist's interpreting the patient's self-deception in a way that the patient can understand. Occasionally, the therapist will encounter outright lies during the course of psychotherapy. If handled correctly by the therapist, such lies can be very meaningful and useful for therapeutic purposes. They do, however, tend to engender considerable emotional responses within the therapist.

In this chapter, I focus on the meager information available about treating persons who are habitual liars and those who live lives of deception—the impostors. I briefly consider issues related to deceit that occur in the context of psychotherapy, lies among substance abusers, the importance of family secrets, and how to deal with the lies of children.

Treatment of Habitual Lying

Lying is, to a very large extent, an ego-syntonic activity. That is, lying does not cause much distress to the liar unless the lie results in negative consequences. For example, a store clerk might not feel guilty lying about the availability of merchandise but might be upset about losing a customer if the lie is detected. Because lying may be a means of protecting the ego and (as is further developed in Chapters 13 and 14) is closely related to self-deception, habitual liars rarely go to a psychiatrist or psychologist (of their own initiative) with a request for help. Almost inevitably, they are coerced by a spouse, parent, or employer into a treatment they do not genuinely desire for themselves.

The first task for the clinician is to complete a comprehensive evaluation. The clinician must determine whether any underlying cerebral dysfunction or learning disability is evident, and if so, whether it plays a role in the patient's prevarications. Sometimes, just the new knowledge of underlying brain dysfunction helps the family take a less punitive stance toward the individual and allows a less confrontational style of communication. The clinician's second task is to determine the presence or absence of comorbid psychiatric syndromes that may facilitate the lying behavior; if present, these conditions must be treated. Third, successful treatment requires establishing rapport and developing a therapeutic alliance. As I discuss below, this does not necessarily mean a frontal attack on the lying behavior. Because lying is a social phenomenon, the spouse or other family members may also need to be involved in the treatment plan.

The two following brief clinical cases illustrate some of the issues related to treating the habitual liar.

■ The Elusive College Student

Spencer, a 20-year-old college student, was referred for psychotherapy after his parents learned that he had repeatedly lied to them
about his college activities. He had habitually failed to attend class,
complete assignments, or take examinations. He generally dropped
courses at the last minute (rather than fail them). As a result, he had
completed the equivalent of only one semester at the end of 2 years
attended at three separate universities.

Spencer's father was a highly successful businessman who had
a golden touch; every enterprise he started made money. He was a
demanding perfectionist and expected his charming, handsome,
and intellectually gifted son to follow in his footsteps. Spencer's
mother was preoccupied with the petty politics of the country club.
Despite his family's financial and social position and his own innate capabilities, Spencer had low self-esteem. He also believed that
there was no way he could match his father's accomplishments or
meet his father's expectations. Thus, he lied about school, the girls
he dated, athletic accomplishments, and whatever else was needed
to maintain the image of the role he was expected to fulfill.

Spencer, although not an eager candidate for psychotherapy,
was a cooperative patient who kept his appointments. The therapist
took a nonconfrontational stance, often listening to fantasies of personal accomplishment and stories of his family's wealth and power.
Interspersed were Spencer's more realistic concerns about the anxieties of dating and how to study for classes. Spencer took a part-time
job in the college library and received praise from the therapist for
his initiative and the quality of his work. The therapist regarded
this job and other new independent behaviors as necessary steps for
Spencer to define himself as a separate person and to nurture his
growing self-esteem.

During an unfortunate visit from Spencer's parents, they subtly demeaned his part-time job and critically questioned why he was
not making greater progress in psychotherapy. Shortly thereafter,
Spencer dropped out of psychotherapy (passively, by missing scheduled appointments) and, at last contact by telephone, was planning
to attend yet a different college.

Psychotherapy can be laboriously slow when low self-esteem is
the core issue underlying compulsive lying. The lengthy but suc-

cessful analysis of "Tom" reported by Dithrich (1991) illustrates the need for therapy to provide space for growth and development of the personality as a whole. Kohut (1984) emphasized the need for a noncondemning, empathetic therapeutic approach and suggested that the lies told during treatment may represent efforts of the patient to assert independence in an exploratory manner.

■ The Henpecked Husband

The complaints that brought Kendall into a psychiatrist's office were, on the surface, similar to those of Freddy (see Chapter 7). Kendall presented himself for treatment at the insistence of his wife, Patricia, who had stated that she would leave him if he did not stop lying. Their marriage had begun with his statement that he had paid off the balance on her engagement ring; in fact, he had used that credit line to finance the expensive honeymoon that she had demanded. He had repeatedly lied (in response to her numerous questions) about things such as how much money he had spent for lunch, clothing, and sundries. Furthermore, she would leave him lists of chores to do around the house and become angry when he lied about having completed them. Kendall lied about almost anything she asked, including where he had been when he was late getting home for dinner. Patricia—an aspiring lawyer working as a legal secretary—would make a case about each of his falsehoods and grill him mercilessly about his deceit. She finally concluded that he was a "compulsive liar" and "sent" him for psychiatric treatment.

As a child and adolescent, Kendall had faced similar controlling behavior from his father, an overbearing retired military officer. He had responded in the same way, lying about completing homework assignments and household chores. He lied even though his father would ultimately discover the truth and become angry. Kendall would do almost anything to avoid direct confrontation or exposing himself publicly. He shunned social events for fear of making a fool of himself. He avoided public speaking, even speaking up in his Sunday school class, for fear that he would humiliate himself. He even had difficulty saying "no" to salesclerks and at times found himself buying things he really did not want or need. It is important to note that Kendall did not lie in all aspects of his life. He was a long-standing, loyal, and honest employee at a medium-sized accounting firm. His friends, with whom he could be more relaxed, liked his easygoing manner.

Kendall's condition was diagnosed as social phobia (avoidance of unfamiliar social situations and a fear of humiliation); his lying was one way to avoid painful confrontations with other people. Following his psychiatric evaluation, Kendall began behavior therapy with the goal of reducing his anxiety in social situations. His treatment proved successful, and after he had gained an ability to handle confrontation, he and Patricia were referred for marital therapy. During a joint meeting with the therapist, he was able to tell Patricia that he would no longer accept her controlling behavior and—later, when she would not modify her behavior—that he wanted out of the marriage. Kendall's "compulsive lying" was relatively circumscribed, and he learned to modify his behavior. However, realistically, he remains at risk for relapse into lying behavior if certain situations in his life recur.

Summary of Case Examples

These case studies (and the others in this text) show that lying is not a simple disorder with one single cause. Rather, it has many etiologies, and many factors may contribute to the deceitful behavior of any individual. Thus, treatment must be tailored to the individual need of the patient (Davidoff 1942; Healy and Healy 1915). In the case of Kendall, it appeared that his lying was closely linked to his social phobia and his fears of interpersonal confrontation. Relatively brief behavioral and marital therapy was effective in reducing his repeated lying in one situation, to his wife.

Spencer's lying was closely related to issues concerning his pervasive sense of low self-esteem. The treatment of the person with low self-esteem is necessarily long and arduous. Unfortunately, Spencer's family was too impatient to allow maturity and personal differentiation to evolve through the process of extended psychotherapy. Such treatment was effective for Tom (Dithrich 1991).

The Therapist as Lie Detector

Most psychotherapists accept, without much question, the veracity of their patients' statements. Doing so permits greater empathy, and the exact truth is often not regarded as important as what the patient feels at the moment. I discussed the potential ill effects on a third party of this traditional approach in Chapter 9, with the recommendation that the therapist remain neutral about the truthfulness of a patient's statements. Nonetheless, the question of whether a patient is lying is occasionally raised, and the therapist may need to judge the truthfulness of a statement.

Othmer and Othmer (1994) detailed severe nonverbal signals that may suggest deception. These signs were originally described by Ekman and colleagues and are discussed in Chapter 10. The Othmers also described "cross-examination" as an interview technique designed to trip the liar. I believe that these methods of lie detection may, on occasion, be used to identify liars in consultations or forensic evaluations, but they should not be applied to the vast majority of clinical situations in psychotherapy. Overt lies are not the central problem for the psychotherapist; rather, the therapist must address selective memories, distortions, and self-deceptions that create misrepresentations. Even when the patient is engaged in overt prevarications, the therapist's skill at detecting lies is unlikely to be much better than chance. Ekman and O'Sullivan (1991) found that only about 12% of psychiatrists had a high rate of successful lie detection. Most people—including psychiatrists—who regard themselves as experts at catching lies are, in fact, deceiving themselves (see Chapters 10 and 11).

Lies During Psychotherapy

Patients frequently lie during the course of psychotherapy, even when they have not been identified as pathological liars. Weinshel (1979), Blum (1983), and Billig (1991) have provided examples of how lies told during therapy may serve as "screens" to disguise underlying secrets.

Billig (1991) reported a fascinating case history of a woman who, for several months during psychotherapy, fabricated a story of her mother's terminal cancer and death. In her therapy hours, she described details of the funeral and helping her father find housekeeping assistance; in fact, no death had occurred. The fabrication appeared to be a way for the patient to continue psychotherapy (avoid separation from the therapist) and, in a displaced manner, deal with the real loss of her husband by divorce. Much like a dream, the lie can be analyzed for its meaning, both in its content and in its relationship to the therapist. As noted by Deutsch (1921/1982) and Blum (1983), the lie may reveal as much as it conceals.

Kernberg (1975) emphasized the importance of lies during therapy as impediments to therapy. He proposed a vigorous interpretive intervention because he viewed lying as interfering with the psychotherapeutic approach to all other problems. Furthermore, he suggests that lying indicates a basic hopelessness and unavailability for authentic human relationships. Kernberg's view of lying during therapy implies that the lies represent an aggressive assault on the therapist and the therapeutic process; the lies must be addressed in order to establish or reestablish a therapeutic alliance.

O'Shaughnessy (1990) described this phenomenon of experiencing a patient's lies as an assault in her reports of the psychoanalysis of two habitual liars. Her own feelings were provoked by the behavior of one the patients: "His lies were delivered tauntingly to provoke me to get out of control. Call him a liar and moralize at him. I had to struggle hard to hold an analytic stance and keep my focus on the experiences received as he lied to me" (pp. 189–190). O'Shaughnessy went on to say, "For L. and M., their habitual lying has the meaning of an omnipotent tongue or penis which opens their objects to their entry and control and solves their anxieties and sufferings with a sadomasochistic excitement" (pp. 192–193).

The lies of a less-disturbed patient can be used as grist for the psychotherapy mill. The lies can be analyzed in terms of their symbolic meanings (what they say about the patient) and their transferential meanings (what they say about the patient's feelings toward the therapist). Because a patient's lies often stir up feelings in the therapist, the therapist must be vigilant. When the therapist analyzes his or her own feelings (rather than reacting to them with a verbal attack on the patient), the feelings can be very useful in understanding the patient's need for deceit in interpersonal relationships.

When treating pseudologia fantastica or pathological lying that serves to protect very low self-esteem, vigorous confrontation (or even overt acknowledgment) of the lie is rarely therapeutic and is often counterproductive. These fragile persons have such severe ego defects that the lies serve a needed protective function. A nonconfrontational approach is much more effective in the long run.

Treatment of Substance Abuse and Impulse Control Disorders

The lying that occurs in persons with substance abuse problems, impulse control disorders, or severe personality disorders cannot be addressed as a solitary symptom. The lying and self-deceit of these persons is part of their overall lifestyle and is intertwined with their basic underlying psychiatric disorders. Their lying must be treated as part of the overall picture. These persons cannot control their impulses and tend to be very noncompliant with any proposed treatment plan; in fact, they often deny that they have a problem. For example, Lisa (see Chapter 7) dropped out of therapy as soon as the external pressures (such as court-mandated treatment) abated. Dan (see Chapter 7) also never acknowledged that he was an alcoholic, and he never sought help until he became depressed after losing his job.

The treatment of persons with substance abuse and impulse control disorders must be more vigorous and confrontational than is usually possible in individual outpatient psychotherapy. Confrontation in individual therapy may increase anxiety and provoke acting-out behaviors (the very reason for which treatment was indicated). However, failing to confront the lying and associated behaviors allows them to be denied and perpetuated, causing damage to the person and those around him or her. A more effective alternative to individual psychotherapy is group work, particularly Alcoholics Anonymous (AA), Narcotics Anonymous, Gamblers Anonymous, and similar organizations. These groups provide a vehicle that combines support with confrontation. Groups affiliated with these organizations meet frequently all across the United States (excellent for people whose work involves travel) and provide a built-in social support system.

"Twelve-step" programs encourage the individual to come to grips with denial and dishonest behaviors that have hurt other people. The "big book" (Alcoholics Anonymous World Services 1976) makes numerous references to the typical dishonesty and lies of the alcoholic patient, particularly in reference to drinking. The AA programs emphasize the alcoholic individual's need to discard any self-deceptions and to be vigorously honest with other people. AA members are also required to make amends to others who have been harmed (often lied to) in the past, unless such amends might injure the wronged party; for example, disclosure of a long-past extramarital affair.

Other 12-step programs—such as Gamblers Anonymous, Sexual Addicts Anonymous, and Narcotics Anonymous—use similar approaches. The process of self-examination and confrontation by peers, combined with social support, provides the core therapeutic experience for the participants in these organizations. Exploring various forms of deceit is always high on the agenda.

Pharmacological treatment of pathological lying might also be considered. Medications are not likely to change a behavior, but if there is evidence of an impulse control disorder, pharmacological treatment may be useful. The selective serotonin reuptake inhibitors (SSRIs), such as Prozac, Zoloft, or Luvox, have been demonstrated to be useful in treating these disorders (McElroy et al. 1992). In my experience of prescribing these medications for patients with impulsive pathological lying, SSRIs have shown modest (subjectively rated) success.

Treatment of Imposture and Munchausen Syndrome

Little has been written about treating nonmedical impostors. When apprehended, they have generally been regarded as criminals or persons with severe personality disorders who are beyond help. A few patients with Munchausen syndrome have received psychiatric treatment. In general, therapeutic results have been limited to symptomatic remission during the time that the patient receives supportive, nonconfrontational psychotherapy. With this treatment approach, the patient may receive enough attention and emotional support to obviate the acute need for disease simulation (Eisendrath 1995). If the therapist is too confrontational or permits too much closeness in the relationship, there may be an intolerable increase in anxiety, and the patient may "act out," flee treatment, and resume the Munchausen career (M. D. Feldman and Ford 1994; Ford 1973, 1982, 1983). These patients are too psychologically damaged and too fragile for any prolonged close interpersonal relationship or insightful investigation of their psyches. Treatment techniques that include close legal controls (such as a guardianship or legal incarceration) and a behavior modification approach may be more useful in limiting their hospital admissions (McFarland et al. 1983; Yassa 1978).

Like those people with Munchausen syndrome, individuals with simple factitious disorder or Munchausen syndrome by proxy are only occasionally seen in psychiatric treatment. They may exhibit a remission of their disease-simulating behaviors during treatment, but such remission must not be regarded as a cure. Rather, the attention (nurturing) received while in psychotherapy may only reduce the need to seek the sick role by simulating or producing a physical disease. These patients remain at high risk for resuming their previous behaviors when support is no longer readily available to them.

Secrets and Family Therapy

Dealing with secrets is a major issue in family therapy. A family secret may serve a positive function, such as increased bonding through private language or jokes. Often, however, a family secret—particularly one that is not shared by all members of the family—decreases communication and intimacy, leading to dysfunction in the family. The types of secrets that are often withheld from some family members include sexual issues, psychiatric illness, substance abuse, adoption, and knowledge of a suicide. The family as a whole may protect a secret, such as a parent's alcoholism, in an attempt to maintain structural integrity. The family may invest considerable energy in keeping the secret and maintaining a false front. As noted by Sir Francis Bacon (1908) and echoed by contemporary family therapists (Lerner 1993; Pittman 1989; Webster 1991; Weingarten 1993), secrets are attended and protected by lies. Thus, the psychological environment of the dysfunctional family may promote the development of lying as a coping mechanism for its members.

Therapists differ on the degree to which secrets should be disclosed (in order to promote intimacy and communications) or respected (in order to protect privacy and individuation) (Weingarten 1993). Some secrets must be revealed—in particular, those secrets that hurt the secret-keeper or other persons (e.g., substance abuse or incest) (Krestan and Bepko 1993). The art and skill of the family therapist are in knowing which secrets need to be disclosed and how to let them unfold in a constructive manner. Secrets can most likely be aggressively revealed as a means to express anger and inflict pain, despite the rationalization of improving communication through "honesty" (Lerner 1993).

Therapeutic Interventions for the Lying Child

All children lie. How does a parent deal with "normal lying"? When should a parent seek help for persistent lying? Neither question has an absolute answer because of the existence of a wide range of cultural norms and effective parenting styles. Even professional opinions are generally based on personal experience. There are scarce empirical data on which to base recommendations, and the following suggestions should be viewed only as rough guidelines.

The lie told by a young child is often a mixture of conscious prevarication and fantasy. Rather than either accepting the "lie" as cute or punishing the child for it, the parent might strive to help the child clarify reality. In one situation, a 5-year-old daughter of divorced parents told her father that she wanted a television set in her room at his house, just like the one she had in her room at her mother's house. The father, fairly sure that she did not have a television at her mother's house, responded with, "You mean to say that you would like to have a television set in your room at your mother's house, and one here too?" The girl immediately answered in the affirmative, and the issue was quickly dropped.

In latency and adolescence, the child clearly knows that he or she is lying. A discussion of the potential effects of the lie in question, and appropriate punishment (if indicated), may be the best intervention. A philosophical discourse on the evils of lying is not likely to be effective and may instead be regarded as hypocritical. As noted above, severe punishment may increase the probability of future lying. Also, if parents wish to decrease the frequency of lies, they must be prepared to hear some things that they would rather not know!

Persistent lying must be dealt with directly. Because it is a risk factor for other forms of misconduct, both in the present and the future, such lying is an indication for professional evaluation. There is no single treatment for pathological lying, and therapeutic interventions must be tailored to the individual. It is important to note the finding of Stouthamer-Loeber and Loeber (1986) that lying is often associated with absent parenting. Therefore, persistent lying can be an indication that more parental involvement is required.

Summary

Relatively few patients seek treatment for the express purpose of requesting help for lying. Even so, the problem of deceit is of ongoing concern to the psychotherapist. Persons who have problems with impulse control or substance abuse are especially prone to misrepresent aspects of their lives, as are those individuals with personality disorders.

Therapeutic approaches to the deceitful patient must be individualized because lying tends to be only one part of the patient's matrix of symptoms. For patients whose self-esteem is very fragile, nonconfrontational techniques are preferable. In contrast, persons with substance abuse or impulse control problems (e.g., pathological gambling) are best helped by groups such as AA or Gamblers Anonymous that provide settings that combine confrontation with group support. Some lies that occur within therapy are best handled in the same way as dreams because the lies may reveal more than they hide.

Although some secrets may strengthen family bonds, others are destructive. A family with harmful secrets becomes destructive, and individuals may turn to lying as a coping mechanism. Family therapists must discern which secrets should be revealed and must ensure that these secrets are disclosed in a constructive manner.

We raise our children to be truthful but find that they lie. How do we help them, and ourselves, to communicate with others more effectively? What is the difference between maladaptive secrecy and a legitimate need for privacy? Secrets, self-deception, and lies are facts of life and, accordingly, must be the stuff of which psychotherapy is made.

Chapter 13

Effects of Deception

Convictions are more dangerous enemies of truth than lies.

—Nietzsche

We presume that information is an advantage that results in an increased mastery of the environment and more power over competitors. For those who subscribe to this logic, self-deceit (lying to oneself) would appear to be self-defeating. How, then, could having inaccurate information be beneficial? In the following discussion, I explore this apparent paradox and investigate both the positive and negative effects of deceiving others.

Self-Deception and Self-Esteem

Why do we provide ourselves with false information? In fact, a major thrust of psychoanalysis as a therapeutic technique has been to increase an individual's insight, to bring that which was previously buried in the unconscious to the surface. It sounds heretical to suggest that self-deception might help regulate self-esteem and promote mental health, yet the data that support this suggestion are robust.

Alloy and Abramson (1979) found that nondepressed people, in contrast to depressed people, delude themselves about the amount of control that they have over situations. These investigators used an experiment in which the actual control of a series of games was secretly manipulated by the investigators. If the result of the games was favorable, nondepressed subjects overestimated their responsibility for the result. If the results were not favorable, nondepressed subjects assessed their degree of control as much less than it actually was. In contrast, depressed patients were much more consistently accurate in their assessments of their degree of control.

The authors suggest that this bias—seeing oneself as responsible for good results but not for bad results—may be an adaptive mechanism to maintain or enhance self-esteem. They also note that it is tempting to regard the problem of depressed persons not as having a negative ("depressogenic") cognitive state but rather as having an absence of a nondepressive cognitive bias (Alloy and Abramson 1979). In other words, the depressed person's view of the world is more accurate than that of a nondepressed individual. Further work by Alloy and Abramson (1982) confirmed that nondepressed subjects had a greater belief (self-deception) in their control of the outcome of a random event than did depressed subjects, who were able to judge the control of the situation in a more realistic manner.

Additional evidence for the proposal that nondepressed people deceive themselves more than depressed people comes from the work of Lewinsohn and colleagues (1980), who found that depressed subjects consistently had more accurate appraisals of their effect on other people than did the nondepressed research subjects. Nondepressed subjects perceived themselves more positively than others saw them; depressed subjects saw themselves, and were rated by others, as less socially competent than the control groups. This realistic appraisal of the self-perceptions of depressed subjects tended to decrease over the course of their treatment. The authors concluded that "to feel good about ourselves we may have to judge ourselves more kindly than we are judged" by others (p. 212).

Sackheim and Gur (1979) found substantial negative correlations between self-deception and psychopathology scores obtained from the results of a variety of self-rating psychological tests. That is, they found more self-deception was correlated with *less* evidence of psychological illness. Furthermore, the relation between self-deception and psychopathology was stronger than that between other-deception (lying) and psychopathology. The authors interpreted their data to suggest that self-deception contributes more to invalid self-report measures than does lying. They also found that lying to others was highly correlated with self-deception in women but not in men.

Evidence for the cognitive distortions of normal persons comes from the work of Sackheim and Wegner (1986, p. 558), who found that "normal functioning" is characterized by a "profound self-serving bias" to their attributions. Healthy persons responded to positive outcomes by saying: "I controlled it and should be praised"; however, they regarded negative outcomes as beyond their control and rejected blame for those outcomes.

Taylor and Brown (1988), in their superb review of numerous papers dealing with self-illusions (self-deceptions), concluded that "the mentally healthy person appears to have the enviable capacity to distort reality in a direction that enhances self-esteem, maintains beliefs in personal efficacy, and promotes an optimistic view of the future" (p. 204). They went on to conclude that these illusions "appear to foster traditional criteria for mental health, including the ability to care about the self and others, the ability to be happy or contented, and the ability to engage in productive or creative work" (p. 204). An individual may admit to, or even exaggerate, areas of incompetence in which one readily acknowledges a hopeless lack of talent. This allows both rationalizations that a person cannot be good at everything and avoidance of potential areas of frustration or failure. These concessions may also lend credibility to a positive assessment about other areas of one's life. Taylor and Brown pointed out, however, that self-illusions may have serious consequences (see below), including failure to prepare for a likely catastrophic event, failure to attend to important health habits, or attempts at tasks that are impossible to fulfill competently.

Lending yet more evidence to the provocative concept that successful self-deception may be associated with reduced psychopathology is the work of Lane and his colleagues (1990), who investigated the relation between defensiveness (as measured by the Marlowe-Crowne Social Desirability Scale) and the presence of a psychiatric disorder. These investigators used direct clinical diagnostic interviews and interviews with first-degree relatives to assess psychopathology in their subjects. They found an inverse relation between defensiveness and psychiatric disorder. That is, the higher the score on the Marlowe-Crowne scale, the lower the likelihood of psychiatric illness.

The findings of Lane and colleagues—that suggest that self-deception and the tendency not to monitor inner emotional states may help protect against a psychiatric illness—should not, however, be blindly accepted as a universal principle of good psychological or physical health. A repressive coping style has been shown to be associated with physiological or behavioral dysfunction, as well as with higher rates of certain systemic medical disorders. For example, Weinberger and colleagues (1979) studied subjects with different combinations of reported anxiety and defensiveness (as measured by the Marlowe-Crowne scale). They measured objective parameters suggestive of anxiety (e.g., skin resistance responses, muscle tension, and heart rate). Repressors who claimed low anxiety actually had more evidence of physiological change than did non-repressors who reported low levels of anxiety. Their work suggests that an individual's perception of distress does not necessarily correlate with actual physiological responses to stress; furthermore, the accumulated physiological reactions may lead to systemic medical disorders such as cardiovascular disease. Lane and colleagues also noted that defensiveness (the repression of uncomfortable emotions such as anger or anxiety) was reported to be a characteristic of convicts who had been imprisoned for sudden acts of violence.

The effects of suddenly removing a person's self-deceptions are dramatically illustrated in two mid-twentieth-century American plays. In Eugene O'Neill's *The Iceman Cometh*, the alcoholic derelict, when stripped of his illusions, kills himself. Similarly, in Arthur Miller's *Death of a Salesman*, Willy Loman commits suicide after his son Biff confronts Willy with his lies and self-deceptions.

Hartung (1988) suggested that self-deception can be used to raise or lower self-esteem in order to create a better fit for an individual's social station, thereby reducing tension caused by a disparity between self-image and reality. "*Self-deceiving up* means raising one's self-esteem in order to occupy a position for which one is initially underqualified" (p. 171). This, of course, can be a self-fulfilling prophecy because it may provide increased confidence if one has the innate capabilities to make the adjustment. If too great a disparity exists between true aspiration and true ability, then the outcome can be disastrous with a resultant marked decrease in self-esteem (narcissistic injury).

The opposite is true if an individual *self-deceives down*. For example, if a highly competent woman marries a man whose self-esteem requires that she remain in a subordinate position, she may deceive herself by adjusting her self-esteem downward as an adaptive mechanism. Such an adjustment may decrease her internal conflict and discomfort, facilitating the acceptance of social and economic security that might otherwise be in jeopardy. This form of self-deception obviously extends far beyond sexism to other situations and explains why some people (e.g., minorities) accept certain roles and inequalities in society. Such people adopt an adaptive mentality: "I must accept my lot in life because I don't deserve any better."

Hartung further pointed out that "lying down" is less likely to be detected than "lying up." That is, it is easier to get away with falsely failing than with falsely succeeding. Other people are more likely to be challenged by the person who is "lying up," because such behavior is often threatening, while the person who is "lying down" is not a threat. Although the forms of self-deception described by Hartung can reduce inner conflict and promote greater social integration, it can be vigorously argued that these deceptions are more harmful than beneficial.

Negative Effects of Self-Deception

As useful as self-deception may be in helping to regulate self-esteem and dysphoric (depressed) states, it also has a far more ominous side. Self-deception can lead not only to the destruction of the individual but also the destruction of others. At the clinical level, all physicians are painfully aware of how difficult it is to get many persons to recognize and act on potentially dangerous and potentially treatable symptoms. Lumps in the breast are ignored, rectal bleeding is dismissed as "hemorrhoids," and hypertensive medications are used for a few days or weeks and then forgotten or discarded. The list is endless because it is a human characteristic to wish to be forever healthy and to deny the possibility of serious disease. All physicians regularly encounter patients whose potentially treatable (even curable) diseases have been ignored until they have caused irreparable damage.

There is clear evidence, as outlined above, that self-deception plays a role in helping to regulate and maintain self-esteem. Is it possible to have too much of a good thing? Fred Goldner (1982) has provided a provocative answer to this question. Goldner proposes a condition he terms *pronoia*, which he regards as the counterpart to paranoia. With pronoia, one has the delusion that others think well of oneself and that one's efforts are well received and praised. Maggie Scarf (1994) humorously described this condition as the *happiness syndrome,* in which people go through life oblivious to life's problems and find "good will and . . . honorable intention everywhere" (p. 29). Scarf noted, as had been previously observed by Bentall (1992) in a wonderfully whimsical paper, that happiness is a relatively uncommon state. In fact, partly because of its rarity, Bentall proposes that happiness be classified as a psychiatric disorder. He proposed "major affective disorder, pleasant type" as a diagnostic category.

Persons with pronoia, as described by Goldner, appear to have deficits in reality testing. They may interpret another person's silence as approval or admiration; an "inflated" letter of recommendation might be taken seriously; and politeness might be interpreted as a meaningful friendship. Goldner noted that current business organizational policies tend to deemphasize the negative aspects of a person's evaluations (reducing the risk of litigation), suggesting that omission is one factor that may contribute to pronoia. Regardless of its causes, the pronoid person may demonstrate poor judgment of his or her abilities and may make serious personal errors; one pronoid person asked the supervisor who had quietly fired him for a letter of recommendation!

Kirmayer (1983), using psychoanalytic concepts, extended Goldner's ideas about pronoia and compared it with paranoia. Kirmayer regarded pronoia as a form of denial that protects a fragile person's self-esteem from criticism and rejection. He suggested that pronoia may come from the persistent grandiose thinking associated with a narcissistic personality. Similar to paranoia, this form of thinking seeks to create a sense of coherence from the chaos and confusion of the social world. Kirmayer actually viewed the paranoid person as a step ahead of the pronoid person because the former has a clearer view of the dark side of the social world and one's own insignificance in the larger scheme of things. Thus, the paranoid person is ultimately less self-deceptive than the pronoid person.

Self-deception can negatively influence the lives of others. Tampa-bound Air Florida flight 90 took off from National Airport, Washington, D.C., in a heavy snowstorm and less than a minute later slammed into a bridge and then plunged into the Potomac River; 78 people were killed. Trivers and Newton (1982) analyzed the cockpit conversations of the ill-fated flight. They concluded that the crash appeared to be at least partly caused by a clear pattern of self-deception in the pilot and insufficient strength on the part of the copilot to counter the pilot's poor decisions. The pilot had denied or minimized the many signs of danger. Similar patterns of behavior have been noted in other airplane crashes, apparently stemming from the pilots' self-deceptive beliefs and feelings of omnipotence and invulnerability. Considering the risk to countless other persons, it is certainly in the best interest of society to take steps to minimize the risks of self-deception in those who are responsible for other people's lives.

The self-deception of so-called experts is important to recognize. As detailed in previous chapters, professionals such as police officers, custom inspectors, and polygraphers have great confidence in their abilities to detect deception; as a general rule, however, they have no more ability than the general public to determine when someone is lying.

Another ominous finding concerns the abilities of so-called child sexual abuse experts. Horner and colleagues (1993) conducted a study in which they presented exactly the same information about a possible child abuse case to eight self-identified child sexual abuse experts. The opinions and recommendations of these experts, which differed to an extreme degree, appeared to reflect prior biases in attitudes about child sexual abuse. To quote the investigators, "The justice system recognizes the inherent fallibility of ordinary witness testimony and attempts to abridge it through its prohibitions of hearsay testimony and conclusionary statements, all of which hold great potential of intrusions of personal bias, prejudice, and self-interest. The findings from the present and previous studies suggest that such judicial cautions be similarly applied to the opinion testimony of expert witnesses as well" (p. 288).

The above examples point to the great dangers to which individuals and relatively small groups of people may be exposed as a result of the self-deception of one individual. In a recent article in the *New Yorker* magazine (Rosenbaum 1995), Alan Bulloch, a leading biographer of Adolph Hitler, was interviewed as to Bulloch's views of Hitler's psychological makeup. Bulloch expressed the opinion that until 1941, Hitler had been cunning and cautious and had manipulated his image to effect his political and military successes. Intoxicated with these successes, with reinforcement by the adulation of the German people, he began to believe in his own deceptions. With a self-deceptive view of his invincibility, he then dropped his manipulations and made a series of disastrous decisions that led to the destruction of the Third Reich.

History is filled with accounts of how the self-deception of one person holding great power—or the mutual self-deception of small groups of decision makers—can lead to mass destruction and a very great loss of human life. In fact, in this nuclear age, self-deception can possibly lead to complete annihilation (Goleman 1985). The following description of the process of "groupthink" outlines how very important, but poor, decisions can be made.

Groupthink: Shared Self-Deception

Groupthink is a term coined by the late Dr. Irving L. Janis (1983), a social psychologist at Yale University, to describe a particular form of defective group decision making. He quoted Nietzsche as saying that "madness is the exception in individuals but the rule in groups." Janis was quick to say, however, that although not all group decisions are poor, under certain situations they can have disastrous consequences—consequences that, in retrospect, could have been foreseen. He proposed that the group process can interfere with the consideration of potential errors or analysis of the risk assessments of a variety of options, including the one under discussion. Janis detailed a number of United States foreign policy fiascoes that he attributed to the groupthink syndrome, including the abortive Bay of Pigs invasion of Cuba, the *Mayaguez* rescue mission, and the attempted military rescue of American hostages in Tehran.

The groupthink syndrome has several features:

- An illusion of invulnerability
- An unquestioned belief in the group's inherent morality
- Collective efforts to rationalize in order to discount warnings or other essential information contrary to the proposed plan
- Stereotyped views of the enemy as too weak or stupid to counter the proposed action
- Self-censorship of deviations from the apparent group consensus
- A shared illusion of unanimity about judgments conforming to the majority rule
- Direct pressure on any member who expresses any strong arguments against any of the group's illusions
- Emergence of self-appointed mind-guards—members who protect the group from adverse information that might destroy the shared complacency about the decision

One factor that influences the groupthink process is the early declaration of the leader's preference on the decision to be made. Group cohesiveness and the need to achieve unanimity override critical discussion by any dissenters. Considerable pressure is exerted on "deviant" group members to either change their views (and so remain a part of the group) or depart.

The process of groupthink has been experimentally tested in mock decision-making groups. Leana (1985) found that the early declaration of a leader's choice of options markedly influenced the group to come to that specified decision. She found that group cohesiveness did not restrict the number of choices considered; in fact, it increased the number of options. However, this latter finding must be interpreted from the perspective that group cohesiveness in this study was defined merely by grouping together students who had previously worked with one another during the semester. A group that has functioned as a decision-making body over time might display different group dynamics.

Groupthink is a common phenomenon in groups of varying degrees of financial power and influence. It can be seen at a service club luncheon in discussions of where to donate money for charitable purposes. It can be found at a hospital board meeting in a discussion of whether to build a new multimillion dollar facility despite the anticipation that health care reform will decrease the need for hospital beds.

Arguably, groupthink represents a dangerous form of self-deception. To meet social needs (i.e., support, acceptance, and approval), an individual suspends his or her independent critical faculties and yields to the demands of the group. Furthermore, no group is truly leaderless. The more powerful and influential individuals sway the group, often deceiving themselves into believing that the decision was obviously correct because group unanimity was achieved. Narcissistic leaders (see Chapter 6)—who need success, admiration, and obedience from underlings and who are inclined to lie under the pressure of their own grandiose ambitions—are particularly dangerous in this type of setting.

Groupthink is more likely to occur when the group is shielded from outside influences. Thus, retreats are planned so that group members will not be distracted by other social roles and so that the group process will, as a result, become more powerful. Clever and manipulative leaders can use the process of groupthink to deceive others, and they may also deceive themselves in the process.

Bureaucratic institutions, whether corporations or government agencies, promote self-deceptions that may result in disaster for many persons. Jackall (1980) detailed the processes by which callous decisions by corporations have resulted in the deaths, injuries, or deformities of thousands of people who used defective products. Jackall attributed this process to the depersonalizing effects of a large organization and to the compartmentalization of functions and decision making. Structural compartmentalization—in which means, ends, actions, and their consequences are divorced from one another—may result in psychic compartmentalization, in which personal responsibility for action is separated from corporate activity. Thus, the corporation or government agency collectively engages in behavior that very few individuals, if acting on their own, would find morally acceptable and compatible with ethical values.

Jackall went on to describe the type of person who is a good fit for the bureaucratic (or corporate) role, stating that the people most likely to succeed in the bureaucratic or corporate environment are those who allow themselves to be manipulated. When people perceive themselves as objects to be molded to fit external criteria for organizational ends, they find it easier to see others as objects to be used. Personal qualities (an individual identity with a clear sense of self) cease to be as important as how well the persona meshes with the organizational ideals. Such people master the rhetoric and vocabulary of the organization, flexibly bending with its needs. Value is no longer measured by who a person is but by where one stands in the shifting factions and cliques characteristic of every organization. Personal identity and values are sacrificed (self-deceptively denied or rationalized) for the good of the corporation.

Many people, in a mutually self-deceptive mode, often relinquish reality testing and turn decisions over to those who appear to be omniscient and omnipotent. This phenomenon is frequently seen in times of economic and political unrest when, in the face of uncertainty and fear, the populace will endow a strong leader with unreasonable powers. For example, the economic chaos following World War I led to the emergence of European fascist states. The self-deception on the part of the individuals of society (it could be interpreted that there was an unconscious search for the idealized protective parent) was gratified by the self-deluded, grandiose ambitiousness of the dictators. Similar examples can be found in recent American history—in the excuses for preparing for massive nuclear warfare and in the transfer of responsibility for the Vietnam War to leaders who "know more than we do." In retrospect, both these situations appear fraught with self-deception.

My clinical experience as a psychotherapist has led me to believe that at the psychic core of each of us is the wish for perpetual life, gratification of our needs for nurturance and protection, and the belief that we are loved—a wish that can be fulfilled by finding the idealized parental substitute. A few narcissistic individuals in their

D. Koresh

grandiosity believe (and convince others) that they are such power-ful figures. Their lies reinforce the self-deceptions of others, with potentially disastrous results.

Positive and Negative Effects of Deceit

The advantages for those who tell successful lies are obvious. They may obtain increased power and wealth by intimidating others or by decreasing their power through misinformation. The liars' sexual opportunities may increase, or they may avoid punishment for misdeeds. In fact, the advantages of successful deception are so great that society attempts to exert many controls, through socialization and punishment, on this type of unacceptable behavior. Unfortunately, the schoolyard ditty, "cheaters never prosper," may represent an ideal rather than reality.

Wide-scale deceptive advertising programs are effective and widely used. For example, the implication that smoking a certain brand of cigarette will make one smooth, sophisticated, and suave has resulted in very successful sales figures. Political campaigns that use innuendos for character assassination have been proven to work; the negative political advertisement has become increasingly more common, often aired at the last minute in a close race. It is also apparent that crime in general does pay, and that crimes which are based primarily on deception (e.g., fraud, embezzlement, forgery, or counterfeiting) have highly favorable odds of risk.

Lockard and colleagues (1980) studied the benefits and risks of a variety of crimes and concluded that the ages of perpetrators of deceitful crimes tended to peak in the reproductive years of 20–30 (deception in animals also peaks around reproductive activities; see Chapter 3). Female offenders are relatively more frequently involved with crimes of deception than are males and are less often involved in crimes of overt theft. Cases of fraud were found to have a low risk of indictment, minimal penalties, and a relatively high potential gain!

Similarly, Bhide and Stevenson (1990) concluded that crime does pay, even if most business professionals are honest. They reported that the retail commodity brokerage business flourishes, even though knowledgeable sources maintain that it wipes out the capital of 70% of its customers every year. Bhide and Stevenson suggested that the self-deception of the customers, who want to believe in fabulous returns, keeps the commodity business going.

Deception is also common in sexual behavior on the part of both sexes. Women who actually have little conscious interest in sexual activity may dress in a sexually provocative manner to attract men (Hollender 1971). Furthermore, they may flatter the "male ego" during courtship in order to maintain the relationship. Men, to obtain sexual gratification, may offer love, marriage, or the promise of financial security. Such behavior on the part of both genders may represent a great deal of self-deception, calling to mind the finding that self-deception helps to make one a much more effective deceiver. Findings from cross-cultural studies of sexual behavior and mate selection are consistent with the hypothesis that underlying instinctual forces may facilitate certain deceptions about how members of each sex present themselves to the other sex (Buss 1994).

The successful lie can potentially increase self-esteem. This occurs through at least two separate mechanisms. The first is that telling an effective lie, one that is believed, provides the perpetrator with a sense of mastery: "Look how good I am! I put one over and I got away with it." This process elevates the liar in relation to the victim, who becomes the dupe.

The second way deception may raise self-esteem is that the successful lie may support self-deception; in other words, if the lie is believed, then maybe it is not a lie. A man may detail his (largely fictional) history of accomplishments, abilities, and power. If others act as if they believe him, he then feels "as if" he were the person he has created. To some degree, if not detected, the successful deception can lead to actual success. To take an example from literature, the Wizard of Oz succeeds because the Tin Man and the others believe that he is great and powerful.

Lying may also maintain the self-deception of another person, making it possible to manipulate that person for one's own personal gain. On the more positive side, altruistic and social "white lies" help sustain the ego integrity and self-esteem of another person. Comments (regardless of their honesty) such as "I love your new hairdo," or "We had a marvelous time at your party," or "You are the kindest person" all serve to boost another person's confidence and self-esteem. Although there may be a latent manipulative quality in flattery, positive social comments do help people feel better about themselves and provide a lubricant for polite society. To quote Mark Twain (1896/1923), "The highest perfection of politeness is only a beautiful edifice, built from the base to the dome, of graceful and gilded forms of charitable and unselfish lying" (p. 363).

Lies also serve people's mutually self-deceptive needs to maintain illusions of beauty, well-being, and romance. Oscar Wilde (1892/1907) emphasized this value and stated that "lying, the telling of beautiful untrue things, is the proper aim of Art." Without license to misrepresent, the art world, including much in literature, would not exist.

The altruistic lie is used deliberately to shore up another person's sagging defenses. Perhaps the most well-known version of this genre relates to the assurances given to dying persons. I doubt whether there is a physician alive who has not, on many occasions, heard a terminally ill person say, "Doctor, tell me I'm not going to die." Usually, and without much hesitation or internal debate, the physician answers, "Of course not, at least not in the immediate future." There is an intuitive realization that regardless of the "morality" of such behavior (Bok 1978a) and in spite of Elizabeth Kubler-Ross (1969) and the death and dying movement, people really do want to be deceived about their own mortality.

The preceding discussion of the positive effects of lying relates to the positive effect that deceit may have in helping an individual cope, survive, or increase power. To a large extent, the discussion has not taken into account the *negative* effects that deceitful behavior may have on others. The following discussion includes the negative effects that deceit may have on both the liar and other people.

People who use deception to manipulate the self-deception of others may be attempting to harness social forces in order to increase their own personal power. They may, for example, feed another person's prejudices, which—as a rule—involve some degree of self-deception. For example, the German people were told that their economic and political problems were caused by Jewish control of the banks and that there was a solution to that problem. A more current version of that technique is laying the blame for the economic ills of the United States on the poor.

Perhaps the most damaging effect that lying has on the individual occurs when that person is labeled as a liar. Deceit provides power when successful, but the unsuccessful lie significantly reduces power. The fable of the "boy who cried wolf" is repeatedly told to children in an effort to socialize them into understanding what occurs when a person loses his or her reputation for honesty. Humiliation may accompany the loss of power that results from being labeled a liar, leading to further loss of self-esteem. This narcissistic injury may devastate an otherwise successful person. For example, Sir Cyril Burt's brilliant career as a psychologist was forever tarnished by the discovery that he had published fraudulent data in the journal that he had founded and edited (Miller and Hersen 1992). A brilliant and creative man, Burt could have rested on the laurels of his genuine accomplishment, but his public disgrace included his removal as editor of the journal. Ironically, Burt himself was the author of an instructive paper on the psychology of lying.

Deceit may be detrimental to society as a whole when it creates misinformation that is difficult to correct. This situation is particularly true when a liar is a respected authority. For example, false or misleading data in the scientific world may take years to correct or eradicate, and many scientists may invest major portions of their time in exploring false leads. Furthermore, the pressures on researchers, both novice and established, to secure grants and faculty positions may tempt them to be less than intellectually honest in their scientific reports. Such behavior is also common in government agencies and corporate offices.

The effects of deceit on individuals can be overwhelming. For example, the dean of a medical school lured a nationally known investigator to his institution to become a department chairman. The new chairman found that the promised laboratory space and financial support for his department were not forthcoming and, to add insult to injury, he soon found himself blamed for the department's long-term and ongoing financial crisis. Another person, a newly married minister's wife, found herself paying the ultimate price of deception. Her husband had denied and concealed his promiscuous bisexuality, and she was infected with human immunodeficiency virus (HIV).

Effects of Lies on Relationships

Clark Moustakis (1962), in an unabashedly moralistic paper, decried lying in general and opined that it made a "true meeting between persons impossible." In contrast, a recent lay press article in *Redbook* magazine (Satran 1993) reported on the different lies of married women; the author concluded that lying, to some degree, was essential to preserve their marriages. Miriam, one of the women interviewed, said "If I told my husband the absolute truth for a month? By the end of that time, we'd be divorced" (p. 93). Another woman cogently observed that what people want in the truth is "all good news" and if "he didn't like something basic about me it would be very hard to take" (p. 93).

Metts (1989) explored deception among college students involved in close relationships. She found that married subjects were more likely to deceive by omission rather than by falsification and that they viewed protecting their partner's self-esteem as a primary motivation for deceit. Students who were dating reported that their major reasons for deception were to protect resources, avoid stress or abuse from their partners, and avoid terminating the relationship.

The empirical scientific evidence for the effects of deception on relationships is remarkably scanty, perhaps because it is such a difficult area to research. It is probable that most deceptions are, as suggested by the *Redbook* article, white lies intended to preserve a relationship. Many of the lies told by college students in sexual relationships also fit into this category (Knox et al. 1993).

One study that examined the effects of deception on relationships found that people "like" each other less in interviews where one person is lying, even if the other person does not know about the deceit (Toris and DePaulo 1985). This outcome suggests that the nonverbal communications—both sent and received—associated with deception interfere with feelings of closeness and intimacy. Similarly, Clynes and colleagues (1990) found that the emotion of love (nonsexual) was blocked when subjects lied in an experimental setting. Burgoon and Buller (1994) found that nonverbal changes (related to increased discomfort) occurred in experimental interviews when one of the participants was deceptive. These authors noted that dynamic changes in dyadic interaction—reflected by factors such as pleasantness, relaxation, and formality—were introduced by deceptive communication, even if the receiver was unaware whether the truth or a lie was being told.

One investigation explored the effects of lies on actual relationships. McCornack and Levine (1990) surveyed a large number of college students. Students queried were those who said that they had been lied to within the preceding month and were in a relationship at the time. The results of this study indicated that the discovery of deception within a relationship tends to be an intense and predominantly negative emotional experience. Factors that influenced the extent of distress included the degree of involvement in the relationship (greater involvement resulted in increased distress), the importance of the information that was lied about, and the importance that the individual being lied to placed on the act of lying itself. In terms of the last factor, a person who places a high value on truthfulness might become very distressed by a partner's lie, even if that lie had relatively little informational importance. Of the 190 subjects in the study, 31 (16.3%) indicated that the discovery of deception influenced the termination of their relationship with the deceptive person. Of these, 51.6% reported that the breakup stemmed from the issue that was lied about, 32.3% reported that the breakup stemmed from the act of lying itself, and 16.1% indicated that both factors influenced the decision to end the relationship.

G. R. Miller and colleagues (1986) reviewed published information about deceptive communications in personal relationships and found that there had been relatively little research in this area. Of interest, they observed that friends were better able to detect deceit in a person than were either strangers or spouses. These authors suggested that "perhaps marital partners often develop avoidance mechanisms to 'shut out' the possibility that their mates may be deceiving them" (p. 504). These authors also observed that being lied to by a close friend or a romantic partner is devastating and that, as a result, the relationship is usually dramatically altered. Failure to detect deception may be a means to preserve relationships.

The effect of deception on relationships appears on the surface to be somewhat contradictory. Experimental evidence suggests that deception interferes with closeness and often leads to the termination of relationships. In contrast, anecdotal information suggests that some deception is perceived to be necessary to protect the self-esteem of one's partner and thus that deception serves to preserve the relationship. This discrepancy may be resolved by the suggestion that the lies reported in the experimental situations were all either neutral or negatively perceived. People who hear what they *want* to hear *do not* perceive that information as a lie.

The Personal Myth

The personal myth, a concept originally described by Kris (1956), has been so intriguing and has captivated so much attention that it has been adapted and modified by psychoanalysts of differing theoretical persuasions, as well as by other psychologists and psychiatrists. As described by Kris, the *personal myth* is a product of obsessive personalities who use significant omissions from and distortions of their past histories to create a view of themselves that screens areas of psychic conflict from conscious awareness. Consequently, individuals create myths or fictions to protect themselves from painful realizations about themselves.

Subsequent authors have provided differing interpretations of the use and meaning of the personal myth. In general, it has been expanded to apply to the universality of human experience (Green 1991; Lester 1986; Potamianou 1985; Swartz 1984; Wallerstein 1991; Wolf 1991). When conceived in a more universal manner, the personal myth becomes closely related to issues of personal identity; our myths are the "stories we live by" (McAdams 1993). A personal myth is constructed in the selective memory process by which we "remember" that which fits and shapes our image of ourselves. We also present ourselves to others duplicitously, playing certain roles and providing selective information about ourselves. Responses from others confirm and help mold the resultant myth. Each person's personal myth is unique and serves to mediate between the internal world of illusions and the external material world; the myth conditions the way we transact our business in the external world (Swartz 1984).

The development of the personal myth is closely tied to the formation of the self. As such, issues related to narcissism become relevant; the personal myth may be used to bridge discrepancies between the idealized or grandiose self and reality. The personal myth can then be used as a shield against painful feelings and low self-esteem resulting from various psychic traumas and underlying fears of inadequacy (Lester 1986).

Myths can have a positive or negative quality, and although every personal myth is unique, some common themes prevail. One common theme is that of the "hero." The hero views himself or herself as rising out of humble origins and, through the strength of personal qualities of courage and perseverance, triumphing over critics and adversaries. A somewhat opposite "antihero" is the person who sees himself or herself as the victim of misfortune, poor circumstances, and mistreatment by others. The victim continually expects exploitation and is thus girded against disappointment and the pain of rejection by others. Each personal myth represents the way one sees oneself in the world, and each myth determines responses to various situations and opportunities; thus, the myth often becomes a self-fulfilling prophecy.

The personal myths of Sigmund Freud demonstrate the points made above. Freud viewed himself as a courageous, objective scientist in his search for new knowledge and the elucidation of basic truths. He saw the established medical and psychiatric communities as rejecting his ideas, and he believed that he needed to struggle against ignorance to establish his theories. Freud lifted some of his ideas, almost unchanged, from Nietzsche, yet he never acknowledged the latter's contributions. In fact, contrary to the evidence, Freud even denied being familiar with Nietzsche's writings. His deceptions (including self-deceptions) were tacitly accepted by his inner circle of "disciples" (L. Anderson 1980). Another interesting aspect of Freud's personal myth is that he used only those portions of the myth of Oedipus that related to him personally, ignoring other aspects of the story (Schneider 1991). Thus, Freud's personal myth was constructed out of selective memory, self-deception, and other-deception. His myth proved to be highly adaptive for him and incredibly powerful in its effect on intellectual history.

To a large extent, the process of psychoanalytically oriented psychotherapy is the examination and reconstruction of the personal myth. People who are "victims"—shielding themselves from further hurt—may, as a result of psychotherapy, reimagine themselves as "survivors." With the latter perception, they reformulate themselves as strong, able to accept whatever may come, and able to face the future with optimism and confidence.

Summary

Lies and self-deception permeate every aspect of our lives; they affect our sense of well-being, help create a personal identity, and determine the quality of our relationships with others. Lies and self-deception can also have disastrous effects on both the liar and others. Overconfidence may lead to poor decisions, and malignant deceit can ruin another person. Deceit in relationships, when not perceived as support, leads to mistrust and destroys or prevents intimacy. One aspect of maturity may be the ability to recognize when and how to achieve these positive effects and the ability to avoid the negative effects of deception by others.

Chapter 14

A Psychology of Deceit: Conclusions and Summary

Human kind cannot bear very much reality.

—T. S. Eliot

We need lies in order to live.

—Nietzsche

In this text, I have examined widely varied aspects of lying, both to oneself and to others. Deceit is a prevalent—perhaps even central—part of life (Elaad 1993) that has received, in relation to its importance, comparatively little scientific investigation. I have proposed a biological approach to deceit, consistent with the theoretical formulations of scientists such as Robert Trivers. We must also consider the sociological meanings of deception (because lying is basically a social phenomenon), as well as its intrapsychic functions. Developmental issues of how we learn to lie and to detect lying are an integral part of the process of maturation.

Based on a review of the literature, it is possible to construct a psychology of deceit that embraces its biological underpinnings, developmental issues, intrapsychic and interpersonal issues, and pathological expressions. Truth and deceit elicit strong emotional responses, and they are consequently interpreted in terms of morality (or immorality); some speculation from a biological perspective on the development of these moral views may help direct future research.

Sociobiology of Deceit

Deceit is a prevailing characteristic and a way of life in the animal kingdom. Camouflage, mimicry, and deceptive behavior serve to help procure a meal for the day—or to ensure survival until the next day. Those individuals who are best at deception or the detection of deception have an evolutionary advantage for survival. Survival allows procreation, and traits for effective deception and its detection are preferentially selected through differential reproduction. Trivers (1985) suggested that the importance of deception and detection is so great that it was a major influence in the evolution of progressively greater cognitive powers in humans and in the structural evolution of the prefrontal lobes of the human brain.

In an eat-or-be-eaten world, there is a high premium for prey to avoid detection and to escape the predator. As succinctly summarized (from Aesop) by Dawkins and Krebs (1979), the fox is running for his dinner, but the rabbit is running for his life! Because the prey is often smaller and less powerful, deception is often an important strategy to avoid becoming a dinner. Thus, in the evolutionary "arms race" for survival, there appears to be some advantage for deception over detection. People also have greater skills for deception than for detection. Experimental evidence indicates that children learn to deceive at a younger age than they learn to detect deception. In fact, most adults remain relatively poor at detecting deception. Professional poker players exemplify the superiority of deception over deception detection.

Deception, although a prominent component of the behavior of almost all animals, should not be regarded as a solitary characteristic that has evolved progressively in increasingly more complex species. Rather, because it is such a remarkably adaptive feature of survival, it has developed independently and evolved many times, just as flight evolved independently in multiple phyla. However, some features of deception in primates seem so characteristic of humans that, at the risk of anthropomorphism, there may be some common underlying biological determinants. Preliminary evidence that lying may be influenced by hereditary factors also suggests the possibility of an underlying biological predisposition toward deceit and the possibility that such a predisposition may have its instinctual origins in species preceding man.

At our current level of knowledge, it is apparent that underlying biological and physiological processes influence temperament, core personality features, cognitive processes, and nonverbal behaviors. It is reasonable to assume that the physiological processes that facilitate deception are influenced by genetic and developmental factors.

The frequency of deception in animals is, to a large extent, determined by the cost-benefit ratio. If there is a high benefit for deceit and little expenditure of energy for the deception, then deception will occur frequently. If, in contrast, there is little benefit to deception and it requires a high expenditure of energy, then there is a low frequency of deceptive behaviors. The same principle holds true for the amount of energy required to detect deception as related to the benefit accrued for the effort. These concepts can be extrapolated to human interactions. In settings in which false communication becomes increasingly prevalent, the liar becomes progressively disadvantaged. When everyone lies, there is little to be gained because the expectation of lying increases the index of suspicion. Therefore, the detection rate increases, marked by failure to respond to signals that are presumed to be deceptive. Conversely, if all (or most) communications are true, and if there is the expectation of such, then lying becomes a significant advantage and is more likely to go undetected. For example, it is easy to ride the trolley in Zurich without paying the fare, but if many people began to engage in that behavior, the need for increased policing of trolley riders would make it more difficult to get away without paying.

The equilibrium between honesty and dishonesty is also demonstrated in business practices. The risk of deception must be counterbalanced by the energy spent in the detection of deceit. Bhide and Stevenson (1990) reported that most business professionals are honest and that one's word is generally taken at face value, despite the knowledge that some people are dishonest. These authors pointed out that if most people are honest, then it is more cost-effective to assume honesty and behave accordingly. Dishonest businesspeople are often not punished, just avoided. If one expends energy for vindictiveness, then one loses twice: the resources that were stolen and the time and energy for retaliation. However, if most people were dishonest, the balance of the equation would shift toward more caution and greater retaliation toward offenders. Thus, in humans, as in other species, a balance is established between honest and deceptive communications. Socialization, by systems of morality, is one method by which humankind modulates that balance.

Pathological lying is biologically and developmentally based. It is facilitated by brain dysfunction or developmental deficits, such as problems in separation, individuation, and the formation of a well-defined personal identity. Poor impulse control, increasingly recognized as having neurophysiological correlates, is a feature of many pathological liars. Pathological liars do not tell better lies nor do they necessarily tell more lies; to the contrary, they generally tell poorer lies—lies that may be self-defeating and easily detected. In fact, skillful liars are not labeled as "pathological" because most of their lies go undetected. Those people labeled as pathological liars have failed to become skillful liars who empathetically read other people and use deceit in a manner that effectively advances their personal needs or fosters closer relationships. Their lies are egocentric, and the pathological liar lacks the subtlety to be adept at the mutual negotiation required to have others satisfy their needs.

Intrapsychic Functions of Deceit

The child's discovery that he or she can lie successfully is a major milestone in psychological development. This revelation allows individuation from the parents, and this knowledge of separateness allows the child to develop a private world filled with personal aspirations, feelings, and fantasies. The child also recognizes that others have private thoughts and motivations. These private thoughts can be shared but only when one chooses to do so. With an increasing appreciation of the differences between oneself and others, there are opportunities for empathetic contact and intimacy that are not based on a symbiotic relationship, as was the case in infancy.

A sense of self develops from the ability to exchange (and at times manipulate) ideas and feelings with others. One learns to manage the impression that one makes on others and to dissemble emotional responses in order to protect others or oneself from unnecessary pain or embarrassment. The persona that develops shapes how one is viewed by the external world and by oneself. Through selective memories, self-deception, and duplicitous contacts (impression management) with the external world, a person forms a personal myth that enables coping and shields against potential harm.

The regulation of self-esteem is closely related to issues of deception. External events that reflect poorly on a person are altered for the internal world through self-deception, excuses, rationalization, and even total denial. Conversely, to feel good about how they appear to the external world, people may dissemble their emotions, provide false information, or play roles. They rationalize and make excuses for their own self-esteem in attempts to look more favorable to others (Sigmon and Snyder 1993). They exaggerate their accomplishments and minimize their failures (to themselves and to others) in order to sustain healthy self-esteem. Ironically, people who become depressed are less able to use this "normal" mechanism of self-deception and tend to see themselves and the external world in a more realistic manner.

The psychic mechanisms outlined above are normal; everyone functions in these ways. At times, however, the developmental process is sidetracked or derailed. Innate biological factors, poor parenting, or overwhelming environmental stressors (e.g., physical or sexual abuse) may interrupt the normal formation of the self. As a result, the internal self may be discrepant from the assessment or the expectations of the external world. Difficulty in establishing empathetic relationships with others can distort information about the self that in normal situations would be self-correcting. One mechanism to cope with the increasing tension is to lie to others and to pretend to be someone other than who one is; another mechanism is to lie to oneself. These responses in the narcissistic individual are distinguished from those of a "normal" person by their magnitude and the degree of distortion. A healthy person keeps illusions within reasonable bounds; at times of great stress, some people may lose contact with reality and may lose the ability to modulate their deceptions. Impostors, including patients with Munchausen syndrome, may defend against certain feelings, such as loss of control, by assuming new identities and playing roles. By deceiving others, they deceive themselves into thinking that they are clever, powerful, and in control.

Interrelation of Lying and Self-Deception

The suggestion that self-deception may have evolved as a mechanism to help one become a more effective deceiver (Trivers 1985) seems to have merit. There are numerous examples to demonstrate that people who self-deceive (and as a consequence are more skilled performers) are more effective in getting their message across (e.g., salespersons, actors, politicians, or television preachers). They appear more sincere and are less likely to display incongruent nonverbal behavior that might "leak" their underlying feelings. Conversely, lies to other people may promote self-deception. A person may lie to create an illusion of being more clever or powerful; in both the content and the process of the lie, that individual may be engaging in self-deception, screening out feelings of inadequacy or rejection. In extreme situations, lies may be used to create a new identity (impostors) or produce situations (factitious disorder) in which the person becomes the center of concerned attention. It is in these pathological extremes that the use of lies to support self-deception can be most clearly seen.

The process of self-deception, lying to others, supporting others' self-deceptions, and responding to their messages with further self-deceptions and lies is dynamic. The following vignette—showing some of the deceptions and self-deceptions of a sales transaction as described by P. J. DePaulo and B. M. DePaulo (1989)—illustrates how deception is an integral part of everyday communication.

> David saw an advertisement for a sporty new convertible. It immediately appealed to him, as did the attractive woman in the photograph who was sitting in the passenger seat. (The deceptive implication was that by owning the car, David would become more attractive to women.) David went to the dealer "just to look" at the car (deceiving himself about his real interest) and was greeted by Sam, a salesman. (Sam had been working at the dealership for 1 week; previously he had sold a different make of automobile.) Sam immediately started telling David about how the car was catching everybody's eye and how the women love it. He claimed that all of his customers (only one to date) had been tremendously satisfied with the car.
>
> When David suggested that he was a "practical person" (deceiving himself about why he actually liked the car), Sam quickly changed tactics. He pointed out the car's safety features, its excellent mileage, and mechanical reliability. David pulled out an issue of *Consumer Reports*, and Sam quickly responded that the car was genuinely safe and practical, and its reliability had only appeared poor because the model appealed so much to the young and adventuresome. He explained that young people don't care for their cars the way they should and get into too many accidents—"it's the drivers, not the car." (Sam's complex deceptive explanation was intended to support David's self-deception.)
>
> David then feigned disinterest and started to walk away, but Sam immediately offered a discount from the price, emphasizing what a bargain it was: "almost like getting a year's depreciation for free!" David then purchased the car, rationalizing that it was "too good a deal to turn down." Despite the car's poor repair record, he kept telling everyone how wonderful it was, self-deceptively believing it to protect himself from the painful knowledge of having made a poor decision.

The above illustration demonstrates the ongoing parrying for position in an ordinary transaction. As a good salesman, Sam believed that he was selling the best product, even though 2 weeks previously he had thought a different product was best. He knew how to feed into David's self-deceptions and when to change tactics. Although David fooled himself about the reasons he wanted the car, David also knew how to work Sam for the best price. Neither party left the transaction feeling cheated or exploited. Each, in his own way, had his needs met. This type of communication is typical of day-to-day interpersonal transactions, whether between partners in the "dating game," spouses, or managers and employees.

People who are told what they want to hear usually do not regard it as a lie. It is generally unfavorable information—or the sense that the statement has been an affront to one's dignity—that is interpreted as a lie. Rick was only too happy to hear flattery about his sexual prowess, but he did not want Cindy to lie about money (see Chapters 1 and 6). Thus, a primary skill in lying is to tell people what they want to hear. As described above, good salespeople (or politicians) are superb at this task. Moreover, lying to preserve another person's feelings and self-esteem is often regarded as necessary to maintain close relationships (see Chapter 13). Few people can tolerate the unadulterated truth on a nonstop basis. Thus, we lie to ourselves to maintain our own self-esteem, and we lie to others to help them maintain their self-esteem.

The relationship between liar and target, as described above, appears fairly benign, with each party stroking the other in order to feel good. However, lying and deception have a far more ominous side. Malevolent people may use others for destructive ends. In Chapter 13, the possible ill effects of groupthink through mutual self-deception were outlined. Corporations and other organizations can collectively produce horrendous problems for their customers. Political decisions can, in retrospect, be unbelievably stupid. Ekman (1992) described how Adolf Hitler, a skilled liar, told Neville Chamberlain what he needed to hear in order to protect and rationalize his policy of appeasement; Chamberlain's gullibility resulted in millions of unnecessary deaths.

Ekman has also described, with some detail, the duplicitous interchanges between President Kennedy and Soviet diplomats during the Cuban missile crisis. Similar to the interchange between David and Sam described above, both Soviets and Americans deceived and self-deceived, but the stakes were immeasurably higher. To ensure that diplomats may be more convincing in their negotiations, the leaders of countries may feed their own envoys false information. Thus, deceit may have multiple layers.

Politicians often play on the irrational wishes of their voters, but they are themselves subject to manipulation. The risk for the populace is that those politicians who seek power are often narcissistic; that type of personality makes them particularly vulnerable to lying and to a diminished capacity for critically evaluating incoming information. Like a good sales representative, a politician tells the voters what they want to hear. However, the relationship is reciprocal, and the politician becomes the mouthpiece for the voters' self-deceptions.

Psychological Perspectives of Truth

It would be ludicrous to presume that one can capture the rich intellectual thoughts of hundreds of years of philosophical scholarship in a few short paragraphs; however, some insights from clinical experience and findings from psychological research seem very pertinent to concepts of truth as related to a psychology of deceit.

Psychological truth proves very elusive. The material world can be measured with a high degree of reliability. However, memories, feelings, and motivations prove to be remarkably subjective and fluid; they are in continuing dynamic interaction. Research clearly demonstrates that one's memories can be significantly contaminated by suggestion (Loftus et al. 1989a, 1989b), and a person's perception of an event is colored by both past events and the emotions experienced at the time. Psychoanalysts have discovered that a person's narrative history, no matter how coherent and apparently intelligible, may have little relation to historical facts; or the facts that color the meaning of an event may have been selectively remembered (Goldberg 1984; Spence 1982).

Each individual creates a personal myth—woven from a matrix of facts, self-deceptions, and misrepresentations to others—to help cope with the exigencies of life and internal conflicts. At times, the exact historical facts are unimportant as an individual strives to find coherence and meaning in his or her life; the psychotherapeutic healing process can occur without strict adherence to actual events. At other times, a person's inaccurate memories or reconstruction of a life story, aided by the suggestions of a therapist, can be devastating to an innocent party who may be blamed for acts that did not occur. Thus, a tension between relativism and reality may exist in psychiatric treatment (Goldberg 1984).

The supposition of an absolute truth and the need for adherence to this truth is very popular. One lay writer stated that the presumption that there was no absolute truth was the biggest lie of all (Slosser 1986). Other philosophers (Fried 1985; Quinton 1985)—at times called positivists or foundationalists—are similarly fundamentalist in their views, blindly rejecting the realities of the psychological world. Fundamentalist views of life, because of their simplistic appeal, have been common throughout history and, in face of the ever-increasing complexity of modern life, are becoming even more popular. Unfortunately, these individuals, in their self-deception that they know the absolute truth, are often only too willing to impose their "truths" on other persons (Nyberg 1993).

As heretical as it may sound, truth and deception are not in and of themselves moral or immoral; they are merely forms of communication. It is how they are applied in one's relationships with others that determines their moral value (Scheibe 1980).

Morality of Deceit

As noted earlier in this chapter, it has been popular to view lying as immoral. Some philosophers have looked to the "truth" as an abstract ideal; others, such as Bok (1978a), have condemned lying and offered its negative effects on human relationships and trust as a rationale for this condemnation. Despite this negative view of lying, it is—as described in this book—a characteristic of all life and a significant part of human interactions.

Some of the reasons that lying has come to be regarded as immoral come from fields of scientific interest (described variously as ethology, evolutionary psychology, evolutionary ethics, and socio-biology) that focus on genetic mechanisms to explain behavior and social relationships (see Alexander 1985, 1987; Dawkins 1989; Krebs and Dawkins 1984; Wright 1994a, 1994b). As observed by Krebs and Dawkins (1984), truth and honesty per se are not favored by natural selection. However, altruism toward a relative may indirectly help to reproduce one's genetic material. If a relative (who carries many of the same genes as the altruist) survives to procreate, then the genetic material of the altruist may also be perpetuated.

Alexander (1985, 1987) proposed that morality may have had a paradoxical origin in aggression. He suggested that cooperation and cohesiveness among small bands of early humans may have helped them compete with, and defeat, other similar groups. Survival for these bands of hunters and gatherers depended on mutual cooperation, trust, and the principles of reciprocal altruism. Lying to members of one's group might adversely affect survival for all, and as a consequence, a strong ethos for truthfulness to fellow group members would develop. Regardless of the validity of this speculation, it is clear that trust and honesty toward members of one's social group are values that are widely endorsed, whether the group is a family, youth gang, or religious order. Values for truthfulness diminish as one's relationships with others become more tenuous; that is, the weaker the relationship, the less beneficial the potential payoff for indirect reciprocation of altruism. For example, a person who would not consider lying to a close friend might not mind lying to an insurance company.

From a biological perspective, parents cannot tolerate deceit from small children and simultaneously provide safety. Furthermore, as an infant, the child is symbiotically a part of the parent; lying or deceptive behaviors represent a rejection of or rebellion against that relationship. The child internalizes the need for truthfulness to the parent and may then generalize that all lying or deceit is wrong. The child's first deliberate lies are rebellious acts, representing the first stage of individualization and separation. In contrast, and consistent with concepts of lying in power structures (see below), parents do not feel the same constraints in lying to children and, in a "paternalistic" manner, may frequently deceive their offspring.

The moral imperatives of truth and prohibitions of deceit preserve the self-interests of power structures. Those in power do not wish to be deceived by those whom they control. As observed by W. P. Robinson (1993), it is the winners who write the history books and define the "truth" of the past. According to Nietzsche (1886/1967, p. 204), "The powerful always lie." To some extent, underlings are controlled by careful management of the information they receive. Thus, governments, religious orders, corporations, and other authoritarian social structures establish a doctrine ("morality") for truthfulness that is motivated by the need and desire for truth from others but that is not willingly reciprocated. The corporate structure demands honesty and full disclosure from workers about their activities but does not provide them with information from closed boardroom meetings and strategy planning sessions. Thus, the morality of truthfulness is promulgated for the general public because it serves to maintain the status quo of the power structure. Lies by those who are in power are rationalized as necessary for the good of the organization; lies by the common person are regarded as harmful to the organization.

Trust is not necessarily the belief that one will always be told the truth. In relationships, trust might be better described as the belief that the trusted person (or organization) will try to avoid inflicting harm. Truth can be a vicious weapon to destroy another person's self-esteem and sense of well-being. Marital partners know this and are careful to respect the essential components of their spouses' self-deceptions, even when it is necessary to lie to do so. In the same way, we do not expect that our government will always tell the truth, but we do expect that it will protect us. Trust is not destroyed by deceit but rather by a loss of confidence that the offending party does not have our interests at heart. Of course, being lied to about some issues is likely to lead to a loss of trust.

Bok's seminal book, *Lying: Moral Choice in Public and Private Life* (1978a), has been interpreted as espousing a position that is close to Kant's for the absolute value of truth (Solomon 1993). However, Bok (1980) has also addressed the need for further multidisciplinary explorations of the effects of deceit—explorations that would include fields outside philosophy, such as psychology, sociology, and anthropology. Subsequently, a number of authors have addressed this need (e.g., Bailey 1991; Nyberg 1993; Solomon 1993). Regardless of whether one agrees with Bok's philosophical views, she clearly achieved her goal of initiating more consideration and active debate of the moral issues related to deception.

Some contemporary philosophers have moved away from abstract principles and have endorsed more pragmatic considerations of the ethics of truth and deceit. Solomon (1993), for example, emphasizes examining the interpersonal effects of lying to determine whether the communication was "good" or "bad." "Deception is, first of all, a way of relating to others and to oneself. Some deception is harmful and even immoral, but some of it is neither" (p. 51). He continues, "Deception and self-deception . . . may not be perversions, so much as they are the very stuff of human intercourse" (p. 51). This view is very similar to that of Scheibe (1980).

Nyberg (1993) asserted that "deception is not merely to be tolerated as an occasionally prudent aberration in a world of truth-telling: it is rather an essential component of our ability to organize and shape the world, to resolve problems of coordination among individuals who differ, to cope with uncertainty and pain, to be civil and to achieve privacy as needed, to survive as a species and to flourish as persons" (p. 219).

I propose, in accord with Solomon and Nyberg, that lying and self-deception are neither inherently moral or immoral. They are inextricable parts of our relationships with ourselves and with other people.

Summary

The search for a psychology of deceit cannot be reduced to just a few basic laws or principles. It is a science in its infancy and, like the subject matter itself, must remain flexible. The accumulation of new data and studies to confirm previous observations must continue.

In the study of biology (the science of life) we find that deceit is prevalent throughout the animal kingdom, and humanity is no exception. Humans take deceit one step further and elaborate on it with self-deception. In the majority of psychic operations, self-deception and deception prove to be so intimately interwoven as to be inseparable. Deception and self-deception serve each other. Furthermore, and of great importance, social relationships influence our perceptions and memories and reinforce our self-deception. Every child, of necessity, uses lying as a means to individuate himself or herself. Lying behavior is taught and socialized to all children, regardless of the paradoxical parental interdictions. We learn how to detect lying from others and how to encourage lying from others in order to sustain our own self-deceptions. We learn that at times it is in our best interest not to acknowledge consciously the deceptions we have detected; thus, we willingly allow ourselves to be deceived and self-deceived.

Self-deception begins early in life, protecting and nourishing our self-image and self-esteem. Self-deception and other-deception help us to shape our external world to fit the needs of our internal world. This distortion of reality is facilitated by underlying cerebral dysfunction, particularly an imbalance between verbal and nonverbal cognitive abilities, or by traumatic childhood experiences. If a child fails to make appropriate empathetic links with other persons (initially the parents), this deficiency is likely to continue in the form of a poor sense of self. In those who lack empathic feedback from others, self-deception may become more extreme and projected onto others in the form of pathological lying.

A few people, by virtue of their inherent acting skills—called "natural performers" by Ekman (1992)—are exceptionally good at lying; such individuals can thrive in occupations (such as politics or sales) that place a premium on skilled deception. Individuals who have this skill and who, in addition, have severe character dysfunctions (e.g., narcissistic or antisocial personality disorders) have wreaked, and will continue to wreak, great damage on humanity.

As we develop the skills to deceive others and ourselves, we also develop the skills to detect deceit. The human ability to detect lies is less developed than our skill to deceive. A few persons do seem to have unusual abilities to catch lies, but the majority of so-called experts at lie detection are, in fact, deceiving themselves about their abilities. We are at great risk when we are too trusting and willing to believe such experts. Most people do not use all of their inherent skills in lie detection, and this process of overlooking another's lies appears to be related to skills in social interchange; too much lie detection may be a social liability.

Deception of either oneself or others—like the instincts of aggression and reproduction—is neither inherently good or bad. With the evolution of the human brain, perhaps propelled by the reciprocal pressures to deceive and to detect deceit, has come the capacity for enormous technological advances. Humans have created instruments that allow for instantaneous widespread communications (either accurate or deceptive) and for methods of mass destruction. The capacity now exists to change the environment and even to alter the gene, the very substance of reproduction. This progress offers the opportunity for humanity to affect social systems and, through genetic engineering, to further human evolution; it also creates the possibility of annihilation. If we are to avoid an apocalyptic fate, we must learn to modulate the instinctual forces of aggression and reproduction and the allied functions of deceit. In the final analysis, it is not lying but mutually reinforced self-deception that poses the greatest danger to the individual, society, and humanity.

Epilogue

This project started with great enthusiasm and the illusion (self-deception?) that new truths had been discovered. As it proceeded, with the review of the published works of many other investigators, it became increasingly obvious that relatively little is uniquely new. The discovery that others have had similar ideas is comforting in the knowledge that one is not alone in the intellectual wilderness, but it is also humbling to find that one is not as creative or as innovative as had been envisioned.

In one of those rare instances when intellectual honesty rears its head above the ugly sea of self-deception, I must confess that others have demonstrated at least equal insight and have often communicated with greater style. It seems that we must continually rediscover the truth.

References

Abagnale FW Jr: Catch Me If You Can. New York, Grosset & Dunlap, 1980

Abraham K: The history of an impostor in the light of psychoanalytic knowledge. Psychoanal Q 4:570–587, 1935

Ackerman BP: Speaker bias in children's evaluation of the external consistency of statements. J Exp Child Psychol 35:111–127, 1983

Adair J, Dushenko T, Lindsay R: Ethical regulations and their impact on research practices. Am Psychol 40:59–72, 1985

Ahern FM, Johnson RC, Wilson JR, et al: Family resemblances in personality. Behav Genet 12:261–280, 1982

Alcoholics Anonymous World Services: Alcoholics Anonymous, 3rd Edition. New York, Alcoholics Anonymous World Services, 1976

Alexander RD: A biological interpretation of moral systems. Zygon 20:3–20, 1985

Alexander RD: The Biology of Moral Systems. New York, Aldine De-Gruyter, 1987

Alloy LB, Abramson LY: Judgment of contingency in depressed and nondepressed students: sadder but wiser? J Exp Psychol Gen 108:441–485, 1979

Alloy LB, Abramson LY: Learned helplessness, depression, and the illusion of control. J Pers Soc Psychol 42:1114–1126, 1982

Alston L: Defining misconducts: parents vs. teachers in Head Start Centers. Child Care Quarterly 9(3):203–205, 1980

Alter J: It's a wonderful lie. Newsweek, July 13, 1992, p 26

Alter J, Collier R: The secret life of Duke Tully. Newsweek, January 13, 1986, p 75

American Psychiatric Association: Diagnostic and Statistical Manual of Mental Disorders, 4th Edition. Washington, DC, American Psychiatric Association, 1994

Anderson C: Pasteur notebooks reveal deception (news and comment). Science 259:1117, 1993

Anderson L: Freud, Nietzsche. Salmagundi 47–48:3–29, 1980

289

Anderson RE, Obenshain SS: Cheating by students: findings, reflections, and remedies. Acad Med 69:323–331, 1994

Andreasen NC (ed): Brain Imaging: Applications in Psychiatry. Washington, DC, American Psychiatric Press, 1989

Appelbaum PS: Memories and murder. Hosp Community Psychiatry 43:679–680, 1992

Arkonac O, Guze SB: A family history of hysteria. N Engl J Med 268:239–242, 1963

Asher R: Munchausen syndrome. Lancet 1:339–341, 1951

Bacon F: The Essays of Francis Bacon. Edited with introduction and notes by Scott MA. New York, Charles Scribner's Sons, 1908

Bailey FG: The Prevalence of Deceit. Ithaca, NY, Cornell University Press, 1991

Bakhurst D: On lying and deceiving. J Med Ethics 18:63–66, 1992

Baldwin D: Who's lying now? The elusive search for truth in the nation's capital. Common Cause Magazine, May–June 1989, pp 32–36

Ballin S, Johnson J: Pending legislation and tobacco industry deception. Circulation 88 (4 pt 1):1410–1411, 1993

Bass E, Davis L: The Courage to Heal: A Guide for Women Survivors of Child Sexual Abuse. New York, HarperCollins, 1988

Bass E, Davis L: The Courage to Heal: A Guide for Women Survivors of Child Sexual Abuse, 3rd Edition—Revised and Updated. New York, HarperCollins, 1994

Benson DF, Gardner H, Meadows JC: Reduplicative paramnesia. Neurology 26:147–151, 1976

Bentall RP: A proposal to classify happiness as a psychiatric disorder. J Med Ethics 18:94–98, 1992

Berle AE: Legal background of communist methods of interrogation and indoctrination. Bull N Y Acad Med 33:645–653, 1957

Berlyne N: Confabulation. Br J Psychiatry 120:31–39, 1972

Bhide A, Stevenson HH: Why be honest if honesty doesn't pay? Harvard Business Review, September–October 1990, pp 121–129

Biddle W: The truth about lie detectors: the deception of detection. Discover, March 1986, pp 24–33

Biderman AD: Communist attempts to elicit false confessions from air force prisoners of war. Bull N Y Acad Med 33:616–625, 1957

Billig N: Deceptions in psychotherapy: case report and considerations. Can J Psychiatry 36:349–352, 1991

Blanck PD, Rosenthal R: Developing strategies for decoding "leaky messages": on learning how and when to decode discrepant and consistent social communications, in Development of Nonverbal Behavior in Children. Edited by Feldman RS. New York, Springer-Verlag, 1982, pp 203–229

Blum HP: The psychoanalytic process and analytic inference: a clinical study of a lie and loss. Int J Psychoanal 64:17–33, 1983

Blumberg AG, Cohen M, Heaton AM, et al: Covert drug abuse among voluntary hospitalized psychiatric patients. JAMA 217:1659–1661, 1971

Blumer D, Benson DF: Personality changes with frontal and temporal lobe lesions, in Psychiatric Aspects of Neurologic Disease. Edited by Benson DF, Blumer D. New York, Grune & Stratton, 1975, pp 151–170

Bogen JE: Split-brain syndromes, in Handbook of Clinical Neurology, Vol 45: Clinical Neuropsychology. Edited by Frederiks JAM. New York, Elsevier, 1985, pp 99–106

Bok S: Lying: Moral Choice in Public and Private Life. New York, Pantheon, 1978a

Bok S: Lying to children. Hastings Cent Rep 8(3):10–13, 1978b

Bok S: On lying. Berkshire Review 15:7–14, 1980

Bok S: Secrets: On the Ethics of Concealment and Revelation. New York, Pantheon, 1983

Bonanno GA: Remembering and psychotherapy. Psychotherapy 27:175–185, 1990

Bond CF Jr, Robinson M: The evolution of deception. Journal of Nonverbal Behavior 12:295–307, 1988

Bond CF Jr, Omar A, Pitre V, et al: Fishy-looking liars: deception judgement from expectancy violation. J Pers Soc Psychol 63:969–977, 1992

Boudreaux AM: Integrity in the National Resident Matching Program (letter). JAMA 268:3315, 1992

Bower GH: Mood and memory. Am Psychol 36:129–148, 1981

Braginsky DD: Machiavellianism and manipulative interpersonal behavior in children. Journal of Experimental Social Psychology 6:77–99, 1970

Brandt DR, Miller GR, Hocking JE: The truth–deception attribution: effects of familiarity on the ability of observers to detect deception. Human Communication Research 6:99–110, 1980

Branscomb LM: Integrity in science. American Scientist 73:421–423, 1985

Broad WJ: Imbroglio at Yale, I: emergence of a fraud. Science 210:38–41, 1980a

Broad WJ: Imbroglio at Yale, II: a top job lost. Science 210:171–173, 1980b

Broad WJ, Wade N: Betrayers of the Truth: Fraud and Deceit in the Halls of Science. New York, Simon & Schuster, 1982

Brown GR, Anderson B: Psychiatric morbidity in adult inpatients with childhood histories of sexual and physical abuse. Am J Psychiatry 148:55–61, 1991

Brown SJ: Recovered memory case ends with $350,000 decision against psychiatrist. Clinical Psychiatry News 23(1):1–2, 1995

Bull R: Can training enhance the detection of deception? in Credibility Assessment. Edited by Yuille JC. Dordrecht (Netherlands), Kluwer Academic Publications, 1989, pp 83–99

Burgess JW: Neurocognitive impairment in dramatic personalities: histrionic, narcissistic, borderline, and antisocial disorders. Psychiatry Res 43:283–290, 1992

Burgoon JK, Buller DB: Interpersonal deception, III: effects of deceit on perceived communication and nonverbal behavior dynamics. Journal of Nonverbal Behavior 18:155–184, 1994

Bursten B: The manipulative personality. Arch Gen Psychiatry 26:318–321, 1972

Buss DM: The strategies of human mating. American Scientist 82:238–249, 1994

Bussey K: Lying and truthfulness: children's definitions, standards, and evaluative reactions. Child Dev 63:129–137, 1992

Cadoret RJ: Epidemiology of antisocial personality, in Unmasking the Psychopath. Edited by Reid WH, Dorr D, Walker JI, et al. New York, WW Norton, 1986, pp 28–44

Cadoret RJ, Troughton E, Bagford J, et al: Genetic and environmental factors in adoptee antisocial personality. Eur Arch Psychiatry Clin Neurosci 239:231–240, 1990

Ceci SJ, Bruck M: Suggestibility of the child witness: a historical review and synthesis. Psychol Bull 113:403–439, 1993

Ceci SJ, Ross DF, Toglia MP: Age differences in suggestibility: psycholegal implications. J Exp Psychol Gen 117:38–49, 1987

Chandler M, Fritz AS, Hala S: Small-scale deceit: deception as a marker of two-, three-, and four-year-olds' early theories of mind. Child Dev 60:1263–1277, 1989

Chodoff P: The diagnosis of hysteria: an overview. Am J Psychiatry 131:1073–1078, 1974

Chodoff P, Lyons H: Hysteria, the hysterical personality, and "hysterical" conversion. Am J Psychiatry 114:734–740, 1958

Clance PR: The Impostor Phenomenon. Atlanta, GA, Peachtree Publishers, 1985

Clance PR, Imes S: The impostor phenomenon in high-achieving women: dynamics and therapeutic intervention. Psychotherapy: Theory, Research, and Practice 15:241–247, 1978

Cleckley H: The Mask of Sanity, 5th Edition. St. Louis, MO, Mosby, 1976

Clynes M, Jurisevic S, Rynn M: Inherent cognitive substrates of specific emotions: love is blocked by lying but not anger. Percept Mot Skills 70:195–206, 1990

Cochran SD, Mays VM: Sex, lies, and HIV. N Engl J Med 322:774–775, 1990

Conrad SW: Imposture as a defense, in Tactics and Techniques in Psychoanalytic Therapy, Vol II: Countertransference. Edited by Giovacchini PL. New York, Jason Aronson, 1975, pp 413–426

Coons PM, Milstein V: Psychosexual disturbances in multiple personality: characteristics, etiology and treatment. J Clin Psychiatry 47:106–110, 1986

Council on Scientific Affairs: Scientific status of refreshing recollection by the use of hypnosis. JAMA 253:1918–1923, 1985

Cramer P: The development of defense mechanisms. J Pers 55:597–614, 1987

Crichton R: The Great Impostor. New York, Random House, 1959a

Crichton R: The Rascal and the Road. New York, Random House, 1959b

Crichton R: The great impostor, in Scoundrels and Scalawags: 51 Stories of the Most Fascinating Characters of Hoax and Fraud. Pleasantville, NY, Reader's Digest Books, 1968, pp 58–93

Culbert SA, McDonough JJ: Trusting relationships, empowerment, and the conditions that produce truth telling, in Advances in Organization Development, Vol 2. Edited by Massarik F. Norwood, NJ, Ablex Publishers, 1992

Davidoff E: The treatment of pathological liars. Nervous Child 1:358–388, 1942

Davis L: A doubtful device. Health 6 (October):92–94, 1992

Dawes RM: Biases of retrospection, in Rational Choice in an Uncertain World. Orlando, FL, Harcourt Brace Jovanovich, 1988, pp 106–112

Dawkins R: The Selfish Gene, New Edition. New York, Oxford, 1989

Dawkins R, Krebs JR: Arms races between and within species. Proc R Soc Lond B Biol Sci 205:489–511, 1979

DePaulo BM: Success at detecting deception: liability or skill? Ann N Y Acad Sci 364:245–255, 1981

DePaulo BM: Nonverbal aspects of deception. Journal of Nonverbal Behavior 12:153–161, 1988

DePaulo BM, Jordan A: Age changes in deceiving and detecting deceit, in Development of Nonverbal Behavior in Children. Edited by Feldman RS. New York, Springer-Verlag, 1982, pp 323–370

DePaulo BM, Kirkendol SE: The motivational impairment effect in the communication of deception, in Credibility Assessment. Edited by Yuille JC. Dordrecht (Netherlands), Kluwer Academic Publications, 1989, pp 51–70

DePaulo BM, Pfeifer RL: On-the-job experience at detecting deception. Journal of Applied Social Psychology 16:249–267, 1986

DePaulo BM, Zuckerman M, Rosenthal R: Humans as lie detectors. Journal of Communication 30:129–139, 1980

DePaulo BM, Jordan A, Irvine A, et al: Age changes in the detection of deception. Child Dev 53:701–709, 1982a

DePaulo BM, Rosenthal R, Rosenkrantz J, et al: Actual and perceived cues to deception: a closer look at speech. Basic and Applied Social Psychology 3:291–312, 1982b

DePaulo BM, Lanier K, Davis T: Detecting the deceit of the motivated liar. J Pers Soc Psychol 5:1096–1103, 1983

DePaulo BM, Stone JI, Lassiter GD: Deceiving and detecting deceit, in The Self and Social Life. Edited by Schlenker BR. New York, McGraw-Hill, 1985a, pp 323–370

DePaulo BM, Stone JI, Lassiter GD: Telling ingratiating lies: effects of target sex and target attractiveness on verbal and nonverbal deceptive success. J Pers Soc Psychol 48:1191–1203, 1985b

DePaulo BM, Tang J, Stone JI: Physical attractiveness and skills at detecting deception. Personality and Social Psychology Bulletin 13:177–187, 1987

DePaulo BM, Kirkendol SE, Tang J, et al: The motivational impairment effect in the communication of deception: replications and extensions. Journal of Nonverbal Behavior 12:177–202, 1988

DePaulo BM, Epstein JA, Wyer MM: Sex differences in lying: how women and men deal with the dilemma of deceit, in Lying and Deception in Everyday Life. Edited by Lewis M, Saarni C. New York, Guilford, 1993, pp 126–147

DePaulo PJ: Research on deception in marketing communications: its relevance to the study of nonverbal behavior. Journal of Nonverbal Behavior 12:253–273, 1988

DePaulo PJ, DePaulo BM: Can deception by sales persons and customers be detected through non-verbal behavioral cues? Journal of Applied Social Psychology, 19:1552–1577, 1989

Deutsch H: The imposter: contribution to ego psychology of a type of psychopath. Psychoanal Q 24:483–505, 1955

Deutsch H: On the pathological lie (pseudologia phantastica) (1921). J Am Acad Psychoanal 10:369–386, 1982

deWaal F: Deception in the natural communication of chimpanzees, in Deception: Perspectives on Human and Nonhuman Deceit. Edited by Mitchell RW, Thompson NS. Albany, NY, State University of New York Press, 1986, pp 221–244

deWaal F: Chimpanzee politics, in Machiavellian Intelligence: Social Expertise and the Evolution of Intellect in Monkeys, Apes and Humans. Edited by Byrne R, Whiten A. New York, Oxford University Press, 1988, pp 122–131

Dickes R: Some observations on lying, a derivative of secrecy. Journal of the Hillside Hospital 17:93–109, 1968

DiFranza JR, Richards JW, Paulman PM, et al: RJR Nabisco's cartoon camel promotes camel cigarettes to children. JAMA 266:3149–3153, 1991

Dionne ES: Gary Hart: the elusive front runner. The New York Times Magazine, May 3, 1987, pp 28–70

Dithrich CW: Pseudologia fantastica, dissociation, and potential space in child treatment. Int J Psychoanal 72:657–667, 1991

Doe J: How could this happen? Coping with a false accusation of incest and rape. Issues in Child Abuse Accusations 3:154–165, 1991

Dohn HH: Factitious rape: a case report. Hillside Journal of Clinical Psychiatry 8:224–231, 1986

Dolnick E: The great pretender. Health, July/August, 1992, pp 30–40

Dujack SR: Polygraph fever. New Republic, August 4, 1986, pp 10–11

Dunbar S, Rehm S: On visibility: AIDS, deception by patients, and the responsibility of the doctor. J Med Ethics 18:180–185, 1992

DuPont RL: The impostor and his mother. J Nerv Ment Dis 150:444–448, 1970

Easser BR, Lesser SR: Hysterical personality: a reevaluation. Psychoanal Q 34:390–405, 1965

Edell JA: Nonverbal effects in ads: a review and synthesis, in Nonverbal Communication in Advertising. Edited by Hecker S, Stewart DW. Lexington, MA, Lexington Books, 1988, pp 11–27

Edwards O: Thrice-told tales. The New York Times Magazine, August 9, 1987, pp 16–18

Eisendrath SJ: Factitious disorders and malingering, in Treatments of Psychiatric Disorders, 2nd Edition, Vol 2. Gabbard GO, Editor-in-Chief. Washington, DC, American Psychiatric Press, 1995, pp 1803–1818

Ekman P: Mistakes when deceiving. Ann N Y Acad Sci 364:269–278, 1981

Ekman P: Self-deception and detection of misinformation, in Self-Deception: An Adaptive Mechanism? Edited by Lockard JS, Paulus DL. Englewood Cliffs, NJ, Prentice-Hall, 1988

Ekman P: Telling Lies: Clues to Deceit in the Marketplace, Politics, and Marriage. New York, WW Norton, 1992

Ekman P, Friesen WV: The repertoire of nonverbal behavior: categories, origins, usage, and coding. Semiotica 1:49–98, 1969a

Ekman P, Friesen WV: Nonverbal leakage and clues to deception. Psychiatry 3:88–105, 1969b

Ekman P, Friesen WV: Hand movements. Journal of Communication 22:353–374, 1972

Ekman P, Friesen WV: Detecting deception from body or face. J Pers Soc Psychol 219:288–298, 1974

Ekman P, Friesen WV: Felt, false, and miserable smiles. Journal of Nonverbal Behavior 6:238–252, 1982

Ekman P, O'Sullivan M: Who can catch a liar? Am Psychol 46:913–920, 1991

Ekman P, Friesen WV, O'Sullivan M: Smiles when lying. J Pers Soc Psychol 54:414–420, 1988

Ekstein R, Caruth E: Keeping secrets, in Tactics and Techniques in Psychoanalytic Therapy. Edited by Giovacchini PL. New York, Science House, 1972, pp 200–215

Elaad E: Detection of deception: a transactional analysis perspective. J Psychol 127:5–15, 1993

Elliott GC: Some effects of deception and level of self-monitoring on planning and reacting to a self-presentation. J Pers Soc Psychol 37:1282–1292, 1979

Erdelyi MH: Psychodynamics and the unconscious. Am Psychol 47:784–787, 1992

Eysenck SBG, Rust J, Eysenck HJ: Personality and the classification of adult offenders. British Journal of Criminology 17:169–179, 1977

False Memory Syndrome Foundation: Frequently asked questions (pamphlet). Philadelphia, PA, False Memory Syndrome Foundation, 1994, pp 1–24

Feldman MD, Ford CV: Patient or Pretender: Inside the Strange World of Factitious Disorders. New York, Wiley, 1994

Feldman MD, Ford CV, Stone T: Deceiving others, deceiving oneself: three cases of factitious rape. South Med J 87:736–738, 1994

Feldman RS, White JB: Detecting deception in children. Journal of Communication 30:121–128, 1980

Feldman RS, Devin-Sheehan L, Allen VL: Nonverbal cues as indicators of verbal dissembling. American Educational Research Journal 15:217–231, 1978

Feldman RS, Jenkins L, Popoola O: Detection of deception in adults and children. Child Dev 50:350–355, 1979

Fenichel O: The economics of pseudologia phantastica, in Collected Papers. New York, WW Norton, 1954, pp 129–140

Fiedler K, Walka I: Training lie detectors to use nonverbal cues instead of global heuristics. Human Communication Research 20:199–223, 1993

Finkelstein L: The impostor: aspects of his development. Psychoanal Q 43:85–114, 1974

Fischer PM, Schwartz MP, Richards JW, et al: Brand logo recognition by children aged 3 to 6 years: Mickey Mouse and Old Joe the Camel. JAMA 266:3145–3148, 1991

Flor-Henry P, Fromm-Auch D, Tapper M, et al: A neuropsychological study of the stable syndrome of hysteria. Biol Psychiatry 16:601–626, 1981

Ford CV: The Munchausen syndrome: a report of four new cases and a review of psychodynamic considerations. Psychiatr Med 4:31–45, 1973

Ford CV: The Pueblo incident: psychological response to severe stress, in Stress and Anxiety, Vol 2. Edited by Sarson IG, Spielberger CD. Washington, DC, Hemisphere, 1975, pp 229–241

Ford CV: Munchausen syndrome, in Extraordinary Disorders of Human Behavior. Edited by Friedmann CTH, Faquet R. New York, Plenum, 1982, pp 15–27

Ford CV: The Somatizing Disorders: Illness as a Way of Life. New York, Elsevier, 1983

Ford CV, Long KD: Group psychotherapy of somatizing patients. Psychother Psychosom 28:294–305, 1977

Ford CV, Spaulding RC: The Pueblo incident: a comparison of factors related to coping with extreme stress. Arch Gen Psychiatry 29:340–343, 1973

Ford CV, King BH, Hollender MH: Lies and liars: psychiatric aspects of prevarication. Am J Psychiatry 145:554–562, 1988

Freinkel A, Koopman C, Spiegel D: Dissociative symptoms in media eyewitnesses of an execution. Am J Psychiatry 151:1335–1339, 1994

Freud A: Normality and Pathology in Childhood: Assessments of Development. New York, International Universities Press, 1965

Freud A: The Ego and the Mechanisms of Defense (1936). New York, International Universities Press, 1966

Freud S: Fragments of a case of hysteria (1905), in Collected Papers, Vol 3. New York, Basic Books, 1959, p 94

Fried C: The evil of lying, in Vice and Virtue in Everyday Life: Introductory Readings in Ethics. Edited by Sommers CH. New York, Harcourt Brace Jovanovich, 1985, pp 291–302

Fuller AK, LeRoy JB: Personality disorders: an overview for the physician. South Med J 86:430–437, 1993

Ganaway GK: Historical truth versus narrative truth: clarifying the role of exogenous trauma in the etiology of multiple personality disorder and its variants. Dissociation 2:205–220, 1989

Ganaway GK: Transference and countertransference shaping influence on dissociative syndromes, in Dissociation: Clinical and Theoretical Perspectives. Edited by Lynn SJ, Rhue JW. New York, Guilford, 1994

Garvey J: Ferdinand Demara, Jr.—his undoing was usually that he did so well. American History Illustrated 20(6):20–21, 1985

Gary Hart and Joe Biden: a surfeit of behavior (editorial). America, October 10, 1987, p 203

Gault MH, Campbell NR, Aksu AE: Spurious stones. Nephron 48:274–279, 1988

Gazzaniga MS, Risse GL, Springer SP, et al: Psychologic and neurologic consequences of partial and complete cerebral commissurotomy. Neurology 25:10–15, 1975

Goffman E: The Presentation of Self in Everyday Life. New York, Doubleday, 1959

Goldberg A: On telling the truth, in Adolescent Psychiatry: Developmental and Clinical Studies, Vol II. Edited by Feinstein SC, Giovacchini PL. New York, Basic Books, 1973, pp 98–112

Goldberg A: The tension between realism and relativism in psychoanalysis. Psychoanalysis and Contemporary Thought 7:367–386, 1984

Goldman B: The prescription drug sting: be careful out there. Can Med Assoc J 136:629–638, 1987a

Goldman B: Fighting back: the search for a solution to prescription drug abuse. Can Med Assoc J 136:745–752, 1987b

Goldman B: Confronting the prescription drug addict: doctors must learn to say no. Can Med Assoc J 136:871–876, 1987c

Goldner FH: Pronoia. Social Problems 30:82–91, 1982

Goldwater E: Impulsivity, aggression, fantasy, time and space. Modern Psychoanalysis 19:19–26, 1994

Goleman D: Vital Lies, Simple Truths: The Psychology of Self-Deception. New York, Simon & Schuster, 1985

Gorenstein EE: Frontal lobe functions in psychopaths. J Abnorm Psychol 91:368–379, 1982

Gray GV: The confidence man. Review of Existential Psychology 14:51–62, 1975

Green A: On the constituents of the personal myth, in The Personal Myth in Psychoanalytic Theory. Edited by Hartocollis P, Graham ID. Madison, CT, International Universities Press, 1991, pp 63–87

Greenacre P: The impostor. Psychoanal Q 27:359–382, 1958a

Greenacre P: The relation of the impostor to the artist. Psychoanal Study Child 13:521–540, 1958b

Greenwald AG: The totalitarian ego: fabrication and revision of personal history. Am Psychol 35:603–618, 1980

Greenwald AG: New look 3: unconscious cognition reclaimed. Am Psychol 47:766–779, 1992

Grinfeld MJ: Impact of Ramona case uncertain. Psychiatric Times 11(10):1,3, 1994

Grinker RR Jr: Imposture as a form of mastery. Arch Gen Psychiatry 5:449–452, 1961

Grover SL: Lying, deceit, and subterfuge: a model of dishonesty in the workplace. Organization Science 4:478–495, 1993a

Grover SL: Why professionals lie: the impact of professional role on reporting accuracy. Organization Behavior and Human Decision Processes 55:251–272, 1993b

Grover SL, Hui C: The influence of role conflict and self-interest on lying in organizations. Journal of Business Ethics 13:295–303, 1994

Gudjonsson GH: One hundred alleged false confession cases: some normative data. Br J Clin Psychol 29:249–250, 1990

Gudjonsson GH, MacKeith JAC: Retracted confessions: legal, psychological, and psychiatric aspects. Med Sci Law 28:187–194, 1988

Gur RC, Sackheim HA: Self-deception: a concept in search of a phenomenon. J Pers Soc Psychol 37:147–169, 1979

Gutheil TG: True or false memories of sexual abuse? a forensic psychiatric view. Psychiatric Annals 23:527–531, 1993

Guze SB, Woodruff RA, Clayton PJ: Hysteria and antisocial behavior: further evidence of an association. Am J Psychiatry 127:957–960, 1971

Gwertzman B: This time Shultz has the test word. The New York Times, December 22, 1985, Sec 4, p 1

Halleck SL: Hysterical personality traits: psychological, social, and introgenic determinants. Arch Gen Psychiatry 16:750–757, 1967

Hamlyn DW: Self-deception. J Med Ethics 11:210–211, 1985

Hankiss A: Games con men play: the semiosis of deceptive interaction. Journal of Communication 30:104–112, 1980

Hare RD: Twenty years of experience with the Cleckley psychopath, in Unmasking the Psychopath: Antisocial Personality and Related Syndromes. Edited by Reid WH, Don D, Walker JI, et al. New York, WW Norton, 1986, pp 3–27

Hare RD, Forth AE, Hart SD: The psychopath as prototype for pathological lying and deception, in Credibility Assessment. Edited by Yuille JC. Dordrecht (Netherlands), Kluwer Academic Publications, 1989, pp 25–49

Harrison AA, Hwalek M, Raney DF, et al: Cues to deception in an interview situation. Social Psychology 41:156–161, 1978

Harry B: Criminals' explanation of their criminal behavior, I: the contribution of criminologic variables. J Forensic Sci 37:1327–1333, 1992a

Harry B: Criminals' explanations of their criminal behavior, II: a possible role for psychopathy. J Forensic Sci 37:1334–1340, 1992b

Hartung J: Deceiving down: conjectures on the management of subordinate status, in Self-Deception: An Adaptive Mechanism? Edited by Lockard JS, Paulus DL. Englewood Cliffs, NJ, Prentice-Hall, 1988, pp 170–185

Haugaard JJ: Young children's classification of the corroboration of a false statement as the truth or a lie. Law and Human Behavior 17:645–659, 1993

Hayano DM: Communicative competency among poker players. Journal of Communication 30:113–120, 1980

Hayano DM: Dealing with chance: self deception and fantasy among gamblers, in Self-Deception: An Adaptive Mechanism? Edited by Lockard JS, Paulus DL. Englewood Cliffs, NJ, Prentice-Hall, 1988, pp 186–199

Healy W, Healy MT: Pathological Lying, Accusation, and Swindling. Boston, MA, Little, Brown, 1915

Herman JL, Perry JC, van der Kolk BA: Childhood trauma in borderline personality disorder. Am J Psychiatry 146:490–495, 1989

Heym H: The impostor patient: Munchausen syndrome with report of a case. Del Med J 45:155–160, 1973

Hinkle LE, Wolff HG: Communist interrogation and indoctrination of "enemies of the states." AMA Archives of Neurology and Psychiatry 76:115–174, 1956

Hinkle LE, Wolff HG: The methods of interrogation and indoctrination used by the communist state police. Bull N Y Acad Med 33:600–615, 1957

Hollender MH: Hysterical personality. Comments on Contemporary Psychiatry 1:17–24, 1971

Honts CR, Raskin DC, Kircher JC: Mental and physical counter-measures reduce the accuracy of polygraph tests. J Appl Psychol 79:252–259, 1994

Hoppe KD: Split brains and psychoanalysis. Psychoanal Q 46:220–241, 1977

Hoppe KD, Bogen JE: Alexithymia in 12 commissurotomized patients. Psychother Psychosom 28:148–155, 1977

Horgan J: Can science explain consciousness? Sci Am 271 (July):88–94, 1994

Horner TM, Guyer MJ, Kalter NM: The biases of child sexual abuse experts: believing is seeing. Bull Am Acad Psychiatry Law 21:281–292, 1993

Horowitz MJ, Arthur RJ: Narcissistic rage in leaders: the intersection of individual dynamics and group process. Int J Soc Psychiatry 34:135–141, 1988

Hulbert M: Lies and near lies. Forbes, September 30, 1991, p 193

Hyman R: The psychology of deception. Annu Rev Psychol 40:133–154, 1989

Jackall R: Structural invitations to deceit: some reflections on bureaucracy and morality. Berkshire Review 15:49–61, 1980

Janis IL: Groupthink: Psychological Studies of Policy Decisions and Fiascoes, 2nd Edition, Revised. Boston, MA, Houghton Mifflin, 1983

Johnson HG, Ekman P, Friesen WV: Communicative body movements: American emblems. Semiotica 15:335–353, 1975

Johnson J: Must this man die? Time, May 18, 1992, pp 40–44

Jones SL: Details of the Nordstrom rape hoax released. San Diego Union-Tribune, May 16, 1993

Joseph R: Confabulation and delusional denial: frontal lobe and lateralized influences. J Clin Psychol 42:507–520, 1986

Joyce C: Lie detector. Psychology Today 2:6–8, 1984

Joynt S: On the wrong side of the bench: the life and times of Jack Montgomery. The Birmingham News/Birmingham Post-Herald, July 10, 1993, pp C1, C3

Kaplan DA: Hung on a technicality. Newsweek, April 6, 1992, pp 56–58

Kapur N, Coughlan AK: Confabulation and frontal lobe dysfunction. J Neurol Neurosurg Psychiatry 43:461–463, 1980

Karpman B: Lying, in Encyclopedia of Aberrations: A Psychiatric Handbook. Edited by Podolsky E. New York, Philosophical Library, 1953, pp 288–300

Kennedy JA, Bakst H: The influence of emotions on the outcome of cardiac surgery: a predictive study. Bull N Y Acad Med 42:811–845, 1966

Kernberg OF: Borderline Conditions and Pathological Narcissism. New York, Jason Aronson, 1975

Kernberg OF: Regression in leaders, in Internal World and External Reality: Object Relations Theory Applied. New York, Jason Aronson, 1980, pp 253–273

Kernberg OF: Hysterical and histrionic personality disorders (Chapter 19), in Psychiatry, Vol I. Edited by Cavenar J. Philadelphia, PA, JB Lippincott, 1985a, pp 1–11

Kernberg OF: Narcissistic personality disorder (Chapter 18), in Psychiatry, Vol I. Edited by Cavenar J. Philadelphia, PA, JB Lippincott, 1985b, pp 1–12

Kerr P (ed): The Penguin Book of Lies. New York, Viking, 1990

Kets de Vries MFR: The impostor syndrome: developmental and societal issues. Human Relations 43:667–686, 1990

Kets de Vries MFR, Miller D: Narcissism and leadership: an object relations perspective. Human Relations 38:583–601, 1985

King BH, Ford CV: Pseudologia fantastica. Acta Psychiatr Scand 77:1–6, 1988

Kirmayer LJ: Paranoia and pronoia: the visionary and the banal. Social Problems 31:170–179, 1983

Kleinmuntz B, Szucko JJ: A field study of the fallibility of polygraphic lie detection. Nature 308:449–450, 1984a

Kleinmuntz B, Szucko JJ: Lie detection in ancient and modern times: a call for contemporary scientific study. Am Psychol 39:766–776, 1984b

Knox D, Schact C, Holt J, et al: Sexual lies among university students. College Student Journal 27:269–272, 1993

Kohnken G: Training police officers to detect deceptive eye witness statements: does it work? Social Behavior 2:1–17, 1987

Kohut H: Forms and transformation of narcissism. J Am Psychoanal Assoc 14:243–272, 1966

Kohut H: How Does Analysis Cure? Edited by Goldberg A, Stepansky P. Chicago, IL, University of Chicago Press, 1984, pp 72–73

Kopelman MD: Two types of confabulation. J Neurol Neurosurg Psychiatry 50:1482–1487, 1987a

Kopelman MD: Amnesia: organic and psychogenic. Br J Psychiatry 150:428–442, 1987b

Kraut RE: Verbal and nonverbal cues in the perception of lying. J Pers Soc Psychol 36:380–391, 1978

Kraut RE, Poe D: Behavioral roots of person perception: the deception judgements of customs inspectors and laymen. J Pers Soc Psychol 39:784–798, 1980

Krebs JR, Dawkins R: Animal signals: mind reading and manipulation, in Behavioral Ecology: An Evolutionary Approach, 2nd Edition. Edited by Krebs JR, Davies NB. Sunderland, MA, Sinauer, 1984, pp 380–402

Krestan J, Bepko C: On lies, secrets and silence: the multiple levels of denial in addictive families, in Secrets in Families and Family Therapy. Edited by Imber-Black E. New York, WW Norton, 1993, pp 22–159

Kris E: The personal myth: a problem in psychoanalytic technique. J Am Psychoanal Assoc 4:653–681, 1956

Kubler-Ross E: On Death and Dying. New York, Macmillan, 1969

LaFreniere P: The ontogeny of tactical deception in humans, in Machiavellian Intelligence: Social Expertise and the Evolution of Intellect in Monkeys, Apes and Humans. Edited by Byrne R, Whiten A. New York, Oxford University Press, 1988, pp 238–252

Lane RD, Merikangas KR, Schwartz GE, et al: Inverse relationship between defensiveness and lifetime prevalence of psychiatric disorder. Am J Psychiatry 147:573–578, 1990

Latkin CA, Valhov D, Anthony JC: Socially desirable responding and self-reported HIV injection risk behaviors among intravenous drug users. Addiction 88:517–526, 1993

Lawson A: Adultery: An Analysis of Love and Betrayal. New York, Basic Books, 1988

Leana CR: A partial test of Janis' groupthink model: effects of group cohesiveness and leader behavior on defective decision making. Journal of Management 11:5–17, 1985

Lear MW: Should doctors tell the truth? the case against terminal candor. The New York Times Magazine, January 24, 1993, p 17

Leekam SR: Believing and deceiving: steps to becoming a good liar, in Cognitive and Social Factors in Early Deception. Edited by Ceci SJ, Leichtman MD, Putnick ME. Hillsdale, NJ, Erlbaum, 1992, pp 47–62

Lerner HG: The Dance of Deception: Pretending and Truth-Telling in Women's Lives. New York, HarperCollins, 1993

Lester EP: Narcissism and the personal myth. Psychoanal Q 55:452–473, 1986

Lewicki P, Hill T, Czyzewska M: Unconscious acquisition of information. Am Psychol 47:796–801, 1992

Lewin R: Do animals read minds, tell lies? Science 238:1350–1351, 1987

Lewinsohn PM, Mischel W, Chaplin W, et al: Social competence and depression: the role of illusionary self-perceptions. J Abnorm Psychol 89:203–212, 1980

Lewis CN: Psychological assessment of an artist and impostor. J Pers Assess 54:656–670, 1990

Lewis M, Saarni C (eds): Lying and Deception in Everyday Life. New York, Guilford, 1993

Lewis M, Stanger C, Sullivan MW: Deception in three-year-olds. Developmental Psychology 25:439–443, 1989

Lezak MD: Neuropsychological Assessment, 2nd Edition. New York, Oxford University Press, 1983

Lifton RJ: Chinese communist "thought reform": confession and re-education of Western civilians. Bull N Y Acad Med 33:626–644, 1957

Lifton RJ: Medicalized killing in Auschwitz. Psychiatry 45:283–297, 1982

Lifton RJ: The Nazi Doctors: Medical Killings and the Psychology of Genocide. New York, Basic Books, 1986

Lippert B: Lying with a smile on Madison Avenue. US News and World Report, February 23, 1987, p 58

Lloyd JE: Firefly communication and deception: "oh, what a tangled web," in Deception: Perspectives on Human and Nonhuman Deceit. Edited by Mitchell RW, Thompson NS. Albany, NY, State University of New York Press, 1986, pp 113–128

Lockard JS, Paulus DL (eds): Self-Deception: An Adaptive Mechanism? Englewood Cliffs, NJ, Prentice-Hall, 1988

Lockard JS, Kirkevold BC, Kalk DF: Cost-benefit indexes of deception in nonviolent crime. Bulletin of the Psychonomic Society 16:303–306, 1980

Loftus EF: Leading questions and the eyewitness report. Cognitive Psychology 7:560–572, 1975

Loftus EF: The reality of repressed memories. Am Psychol 48:518–537, 1993

Loftus EF, Hoffman HG: Misinformation and memory: the creation of new memories. J Exp Psychol Gen 118:100–104, 1989

Loftus EF, Ketcham K: Witness for the Defense. New York, St. Martin's Press, 1991

Loftus EF, Ketcham K: The Myth of Repressed Memory. New York, St. Martin's Press, 1994

Loftus EF, Klinger MR: Is the unconscious smart or dumb? Am Psychol 47:461–465, 1992

Loftus EF, Loftus GR: On the permanence of stored information in the human brain. Am Psychol 35:409–420, 1980

Loftus EF, Palmer JC: Reconstruction of automobile destruction: an example of the interaction between language and memory. Journal of Verbal Learning and Verbal Behavior 13:585–589, 1974

Loftus EF, Zanni G: Eyewitness testimony: the influence of the wording of a question. Bulletin of the Psychonomic Society 5:86–88, 1975

Loftus EF, Donders K, Hoffman HG, et al: Creating new memories that are quickly accessed and confidently held. Memory and Cognition 17:607–616, 1989a

Loftus EF, Korf NL, Schooler JW: Misguided memories: sincere distortions of reality, in Credibility Assessment. Edited by Yuille JC. Dordrecht (Netherlands), Kluwer Academic Publications, 1989b, pp 155–173

Loftus EF, Garry M, Brown SW, et al: Near-natal memories, past-life memories, and other memory myths. Am J Clin Hypn 36:176–179, 1994

Lykken DT: A study of anxiety in the sociopathic personality. Journal of Abnormal and Social Psychology 55:6–10, 1957

Lykken DT: Psychology and the lie detector industry. Am Psychol 29:725–739, 1974

Lykken DT: Reply to Raskin and Kirchner. Jurimetrics 27:278–282, 1987a

Lykken DT: The validity of tests: caveat emptor. Jurimetrics 27:263–270, 1987b

Lykken DT: Why (some) Americans believe in the lie detector while others believe in guilty knowledge test. Integr Physiol Behav Sci 26:214–222, 1991

MacKinnon RA, Michels R: The Psychiatric Interview in Clinical Practice. Philadelphia, PA, WB Saunders, 1971

Marcos LR: Lying: a particular defense met in psychoanalytic therapy. Am J Psychoanal 32:195–202, 1972

Matas M, Marriott A: The girl who cried wolf: pseudologia phantastica and sexual abuse. Can J Psychiatry 32:305–309, 1987

Maurer DW: The American Confidence Man. Springfield, IL, Charles C Thomas, 1974

Mayes AR, Mendell PR, Pickering A: Is organic amnesia caused by a selective deficit in remembering contextual information? Cortex 21:167–202, 1985

McAdams DP: Stories We Live By: Personal Myths and the Making of the Self. New York, William Morrow, 1993

McCarthy J: The master impostor: an incredible tale. Life, January 28, 1952, pp 79–89

McCornack SA, Levine TR: When lies are uncovered: emotional and relational outcomes of discovered deception. Communication Monographs 57:119–138, 1990

McElroy SL, Hudson JI, Pope HG: The DSM-III-R impulse control disorders not otherwise classified: clinical characteristics and relationship to other psychiatric disorders. Am J Psychiatry 149:318–327, 1992

McFarland BH, Resnick M, Bloom JD: Ensuring continuity of care for a Munchausen patient through a public guardian. Hosp Community Psychiatry 34:65–67, 1983

McGivern G: Honor among thieves. Crime and Delinquency 28:559–563, 1982

McHugh PR: Psychiatric misadventures. American Scholar 61:497–510, 1992

McHugh PR: Psychotherapy awry. American Scholar 63:17–30, 1994

McKeganey N: Shadowland: general practitioners and the treatment of opiate-abusing patients. British Journal of Addictions 83:373–386, 1988

McLoughlin M, Steler JL, Witkin G: A nation of liars? U.S. News and World Report, February 23, 1987, pp 54–60

Menger RK: Openness and honesty versus coercion and deception in psychological research. Am Psychol 28:1030–1034, 1973

Mercer B, Wapner W, Gardner H, et al: A study of confabulation. Arch Neurol 34:429–433, 1977

Metts S: An exploratory investigation of deception in close relationships. Journal of Social and Personal Relationships 6:159–179, 1989

Miller DJ, Hersen M: Research Fraud in the Behavioral and Biomedical Sciences. New York, Wiley, 1992

Miller GR, Mongeau PA, Sleight C: Fudging with friends and lying with lovers. Journal of Social and Personal Relationships 3:495–512, 1986

Miller WB, Geertz H, Cutter HSG: Aggression in a boys' street corner group. Psychiatry 24:283–298, 1961

Mitchel AA, Olson JC: Are product attribute beliefs the only mediator of advertising effects on brand attitude? Journal of Marketing Research 18:318–332, 1981

Mitchell RW, Thompson NS (eds): Deception: Perspectives on Human and Nonhuman Deceit. Albany, NY, State University of New York Press, 1986

Modell JG, Mountz JM, Ford CV: Pathological lying associated with thalamic dysfunction demonstrated by ^{99m}Tc-HM-PAO single-photon emission computed tomography. J Neuropsychiatry Clin Neurosci 4:442–446, 1992

Morris MD: Large-scale deception: deceit by captive elephants?, in Deception: Perspectives on Human and Nonhuman Deceit. Edited by Mitchell RW, Thompson NS. Albany, NY, State University of New York Press, 1986, pp 183–191

Moustakis CE: Honesty, idiocy, and manipulation. Journal of Humanistic Psychology 2:1–15, 1962

Munn CA: The deceptive use of alarm calls by sentinel species in mixed-species flocks of neotropical birds, in Deception: Perspectives on Human and Nonhuman Deceit. Edited by Mitchell RW, Thompson NS. Albany, NY, State University of New York Press, 1986, pp 169–175

My Problem. Good Housekeeping 218(3):28–30, 1994

Neill M: Posing as an astronaut was just one small step for flim-flam man Robert Hunt. People Weekly 31:271–274, 1989

Neisser V, Harsch N: Phantom flashbulbs: false recollections of hearing the news about Challenger, in Affect and Accuracy in Recall: Studies of "Flashbulb" Memories. Edited by Winograd E, Neisser E. Cambridge (England), Cambridge University Press, 1992, pp 9–31

Nietzsche F: The Will to Power (1886). Translated by Kaufman W, Hollingdale RJ. New York, Random House, 1967

Nietzsche F: Beyond Good and Evil: Prelude to a Philosophy of the Future (1886). Translated by Hollingdale RJ. London, Penguin Books, 1990

Nordahl TE, Benkelfat C, Semple WE, et al: Cerebral glucose metabolic rates in obsessive-compulsive disorders. Neuropsychopharmacology 2:23–28, 1989

Novack DH, Plumer R, Smith RL, et al: Changes in physician's attitudes toward telling the cancer patient. JAMA 241:897–900, 1979

Novack DH, Detering BS, Farrow L, et al: Physician's attitudes toward using deception to resolve difficult ethical problems. JAMA 261:2980–2985, 1989

Nyberg D: The Varnished Truth: Truth Telling and Deceiving in Ordinary Life. Chicago, IL, University of Chicago Press, 1993

Office of Technology Assessment (OTA): Scientific Validity of Polygraph Testing: A Research Review and Evaluation. Washington, DC, US Government Printing Office, 1985

O'Leary KM, Brouwers P, Gardner DL, et al: Neuropsychological testing of patients with borderline personality disorder. Am J Psychiatry 148:106–111, 1991

Oliver RL: An interpretation of the attitudinal and behavioral effects of puffery. Journal of Consumer Affairs 13:8–27, 1979

Orwell G: 1984. New York, Harcourt Brace Jovanovich, 1949

O'Shaughnessy E: Can a liar be psychoanalyzed? Int J Psychoanal 71:187–195, 1990

Othmer E, Othmer SC: Falsifying and lying, in The Clinical Interview Using DSM-IV, Vol 2: The Difficult Patient. Washington, DC, American Psychiatric Press, 1994, pp 349–384

Pancratz L: Patient deception as a health care risk. Perspectives in Healthcare Risk Management, Spring, 1989, pp 5–7

Pancratz L, Lezak MD: Cerebral dysfunction in the Munchausen syndrome. Hillside Journal of Clinical Psychiatry 9:195–206, 1987

Pancratz L, Hickam DH, Toth S: The identification and management of drug-seeking behavior in a medical center. Drug Alcohol Depend 24:115–118, 1989

Patrick CJ: Emotion and psychopathy: startling new insights. Psychophysiology 31:319–330, 1994

Patterson J, Kim P: The Day America Told the Truth. New York, Prentice-Hall, 1991

Peck MS: People of the Lie. New York, Touchstone, 1983

Person ES: Manipulativeness in entrepreneurs and psychopaths, in Unmasking the Psychopath. Edited by Reid WH, Dorr D, Walker JI, et al. New York, WW Norton, 1986, pp 256–273

Petersdorf RG: A matter of integrity. Acad Med 64:119–123, 1989

Peterson CC, Peterson JL, Seeto I: Developmental changes in ideas about lying. Child Dev 54:1529–1535, 1983

Piaget J: The Moral Judgement of the Child (1932). Translated by Gabain M. New York, Free Press, 1965

Pittman F: Private Lies: Infidelity and the Betrayal of Intimacy. New York, WW Norton, 1989

Potamianou A: The personal myth: points and counterpoints. Psychoanal Study Child 40:285–296, 1985

Potterat JJ, Phillips L, Muth JB: Lying to military physicians about risk factors for HIV infections (letter). JAMA 257:1727, 1987

Powell GE, Gudjonsson GH, Mullen P: Application of the guilty-knowledge technique in a case of pseudologia fantastica. Personality and Individual Differences 4:141–146, 1983

Premack D: "Does the chimpanzee have a theory of mind?" revisited, in Machiavellian Intelligence: Social Expertise and the Evolution of Intellect in Monkeys, Apes and Humans. Edited by Byrne R, Whiten A. New York, Oxford University Press, 1988, pp 160–179

Preston IL: The FTC's handling of puffery and other selling claims made "by implication." Journal of Business Research 5:155–181, 1977

Pyles R: Therapeutic challenges in the treatment of pathological gambling. Psychiatric Times 6:23–25, 1989

Quinton A: Character and culture, in Vice and Virtue in Everyday Life: Introductory Readings in Ethics. Edited by Sommers CH. New York, Harcourt Brace Jovanovich, 1985, pp 291–302

Raskin DC, Kircher JC: The validity of Lykken's criticisms: fact or fancy? Jurimetrics 27:271–277, 1987

Raskin DC, Podlensky JA: Truth and deception: a reply to Lykken. Psychol Bull 86:54–59, 1979

Raskin DC, Kircher JC, Horowitz SW, et al: Recent laboratory and field research on polygraph techniques, in Credibility Assessment. Edited by Yuille JC. Dordrecht (Netherlands), Kluwer Academic Publications, 1989, pp 1–24

Rennie D: Editors and auditors (editorial). JAMA 261:2543–2545, 1989

Robinson G, Merav A: Informed consent: recall by patients tested postoperatively. Ann Thorac Surg 22:209–212, 1976

Robinson WP: Lying in the public domain. American Behavioral Scientist 36:359–382, 1993

Rogers R, Dion KL, Lynett E: Diagnostic validity of antisocial disorder: a prototypical analysis. Law and Human Behavior 16:677–689, 1992

Rosenbaum R: Explaining Hitler. New Yorker 71 (May 1):50–70, 1995

Rosenberg DA: Web of deceit: a literature review of Munchausen syndrome by proxy. Child Abuse Negl 11:547–563, 1987

Rosenthal R, DePaulo BM: Sexual differences in eavesdropping on nonverbal clues. J Pers Soc Psychol 37:273–285, 1979

Rotenberg KJ, Simourd L, Moore D: Children's use of a verbal-nonverbal consistency principle to infer truth and lying. Child Dev 60:309–322, 1989

Rotfeld HJ, Rotzoll KB: Is advertising puffery believed? Journal of Advertising 9:16–20, 1980

Rowe DC: Genetic and environmental components of antisocial behavior: a study of 265 twin pairs. Criminology 24:513–532, 1986

Saarni C: Children's understanding of display rules for expressive behavior. Developmental Psychology 15:424–429, 1979

Saarni C: Social and affective functions of nonverbal behavior: developmental concerns, in Development of Nonverbal Behavior in Children. Edited by Feldman RS. New York, Springer-Verlag, 1982, pp 123–147

Saarni C: An observational study of children's attempts to monitor their expressive behavior. Child Dev 55:1504–1513, 1984

Saarni C, von Salisch M: The socialization of emotional dissemblance, in Lying and Deception in Everyday Life. Edited by Lewis M, Saarni C. New York, Guilford, 1993, pp 106–125

Sackheim HA, Gur RC: Self-deception, other deception, and self-reported psychopathology. J Consult Clin Psychol 47:213–215, 1979

Sackheim HA, Wegner AZ: Attributional patterns in depression and euthymia. Arch Gen Psychiatry 43:553–560, 1986

Safire W: The poly lobby. The New York Times, March 17, 1994, p A23

Satran PR: The lies we tell for love. Redbook, January 1993, pp 56–59

Saxe L: Lying: thoughts of an applied social psychologist. Am Psychol 46:409–415, 1991

Scarf M: The happiness syndrome. The New Republic 211(23):25–29, 1994

Schaller M: Reckoning With Reagan: America and Its President in the 1980s. New York, Oxford University Press, 1992

Scheibe KE: In defense of lying: on the moral neutrality of misrepresentation. Berkshire Review 15:15–24, 1980

Schmauk FJ: Punishment, arousal, and avoidance learning in sociopaths. J Abnorm Psychol 76:325–335, 1970

Schneider M: The Oedipus myth as Freud's personal myth, in The Personal Myth in Psychoanalytic Theory. Edited by Hartocollis P, Graham ID. Madison, CT, International Universities Press, 1991, pp 149–160

Schreier HA, Libow JA: Hurting for Love. New York, Guilford, 1993

Segal HA: Initial psychiatric findings of recently repatriated prisoners of war. Am J Psychiatry 111:358–363, 1954

Selling LS: The psychiatric aspects of the pathological liar. Nervous Child 1:358–388, 1942

Shapiro MF, Charrow JD: The role of data audits in detecting scientific misconduct. JAMA 261:2505–2511, 1989

Sharrock R, Cresswell M: Pseudologia fantastica: a case study of a man charged with murder. Med Sci Law 29:323–328, 1989

Sheehan N: A Bright and Shining Lie. New York, Random House, 1988

Shibles W: Lying: A Critical Analysis. Whitewater, WI, Language Press, 1985

Sifakis C: Hoaxes and Scams: A Compendium of Deceptions, Ruses, and Swindles. New York, Facts on File, 1993, pp 69–70

Sigall H, Michela J: I'll bet you say that to all the girls: physical attractiveness and reactions to praise. J Pers 44:611–626, 1976

Sigmon ST, Snyder CR: Looking at oneself in a rose-colored mirror: the role of excuses in the negotiation of personal reality, in Lying and Deception in Everyday Life. Edited by Lewis M, Saarni C. New York, Guilford, 1993, pp 148–165

Silverman JM, Pinkham L, Horvath TB, et al: Affective and impulsive personality traits in the relatives of patients with borderline personality disorder. Am J Psychiatry 148:1378–1386, 1991

Slosser B: The honest truth about lying. Saturday Evening Post, September 1986, pp 36–37

Smith JH: The first lie. Psychiatry 31:61–68, 1968

Snyder CR, Higgins RL: From making to being the excuse: an analysis of deception and verbal-nonverbal issues. Journal of Nonverbal Behavior 12:237–252, 1988

Snyder S: Pseudologia fantastica in the borderline patient. Am J Psychiatry 143:1287–1289, 1986

Sodian B: The development of deception in young children. British Journal of Developmental Psychology 9:173–178, 1991

Soloff PH, Cornelius J, George A: The depressed borderline: one disorder or two? Psychopharmacol Bull 17:23–30, 1991

Solomon RC: What a tangled web: deception and self-deception in philosophy, in Lying and Deception in Everyday Life. Edited by Lewis M, Saarni C. New York, Guilford, 1993, pp 30–58

Sordahl TA: Evolutionary aspects of avian distribution display: variation in American avocet and black-necked stilt antipredator behavior, in Deception: Perspectives on Human and Nonhuman Deceit. Edited by Mitchell RW, Thompson NS. Albany, NY, State University of New York Press, 1986, pp 87–112

Soules MR, Stewart SK, Brown KM, et al: The spectrum of alleged rape. J Reprod Med 20:33–39, 1978

Spence DP: Narrative Truth and Historical Truth: Meaning and Interpretation in Psychoanalysis. New York, WW Norton, 1982

Spivak H, Rodin G, Sutherland A: The psychology of factitious disorders. Psychosomatics 35:25–34, 1994

Squire EN, Huss K, Huss R: Where there's smoke there are liars (letter). JAMA 266:2702, 1991

Stein DJ, Hollander E, Liebowitz MR: Neurobiology of impulsivity and the impulse control disorders. J Neuropsychiatry Clin Neurosci 5:9–17, 1993

Steinbrook R: The polygraph test: a flawed diagnostic method (editorial). N Engl J Med 327:122–123, 1992

Steiner G: After Babel: Aspects of Language and Translation. Oxford (England), Oxford University Press, 1975

Stewart DW, Hecker S, Graham JL: It's more than what you say: assessing the influence of nonverbal communication in marketing. Psychology and Marketing 4:303–322, 1987

Stiff JB, Miller GR: "Come to think of it . . . ": interrogative probes, deceptive communication, and deception detection. Human Communication Research 12:339–357, 1986

Stoller RJ: Sexual excitement. Arch Gen Psychiatry 33:899–909, 1976

Stout PA, Leckenby JD: Let the music play: music as a nonverbal element in television commercials, in Nonverbal Communication in Advertising. Edited by Hecker S, Stewart DW. Lexington, MA, Lexington Books, 1988, pp 207–223

Stouthamer-Loeber M: Lying as a problem behavior in children: a review. Clinical Psychology Review 6:267–289, 1986

Stouthamer-Loeber M, Loeber R: Boys who lie. J Abnorm Child Psychol 14:551–564, 1986

Strom JN, Barone DF: Self-deception, self-esteem, and control over drinking at different stages of alcohol involvement. Journal of Drug Issues 23:705–714, 1993

Strupp HH, Hadley SW, Gomes-Schwartz B: Psychotherapy for Better or Worse: The Problem of Negative Effects. New York, Jason Aronson, 1977

Stuss DT, Alexander MP, Lieberman A, et al: An extraordinary form of confabulation. Neurology 23:1166–1172, 1978

Swartz P: Personal myth: a preliminary statement. Percept Mot Skills 58:363–378, 1984

Swedo SE, Schapiro MD, Grady CL, et al: Cerebral glucose metabolism in childhood-onset obsessive-compulsive disorder. Arch Gen Psychiatry 46:518–523, 1989

Szasz TS: Drugs, doctors and deceit (letter). N Engl J Med 286:111, 1972

Szucko JJ, Kleinmuntz B: Statistical versus clinical lie detection. Am Psychol 6:488–496, 1981

Tate CS, Warren AR, Hess TM: Adults' liability for children's "lie-ability": can adults coach children to lie successfully?, in Cognitive and Social Factors in Early Deception. Edited by Ceci SJ, Leichtman MD, Putnick ME. Hillsdale, NJ, Erlbaum, 1992, pp 69–87

Tausk V: On the origin of the "influencing machine" in schizophrenia. Psychoanal Q 2:519–556, 1933

Tavris C: Beware the incest survivor machine. The New York Times Book Review, January 3, 1993, pp 1, 16–17

Taylor SE, Brown JD: Illusion and well-being: a social psychological perspective on mental health. Psychol Bull 103:193–210, 1988

Toris C, DePaulo BM: Effects of actual deception and suspiciousness of deception on interpersonal perceptions. J Pers Soc Psychol 47:1063–1073, 1985

Touhey JC: Child-rearing antecedents and the emergence of Machiavellianism. Sociometry 36:194–206, 1973

Toy D, Olsen J, Wright L: Effects of debriefing in marketing research involving "mild" deceptions. Psychology and Marketing 6:69–85, 1989

Trepman E: The oath betrayed: the physician soldiers of Nazi Germany. Harvard Medical Alumni Bulletin, Spring, 1988, pp 28–32

Trivers RL: The evolution of reciprocal altruism. Q Rev Biol 46:35–57, 1971

Trivers RL: Deceit and self-deception, in Social Evolution. Menlo Park, CA, Benjamin/Cummings, 1985, pp 320–395

Trivers RL: Foreword, in Self-Deception: An Adaptive Mechanism? Edited by Lockard JS, Paulus DL. Englewood Cliffs, NJ, Prentice-Hall, 1988, pp vii–ix

Trivers RL, Newton HP: The crash of flight 90: doomed by self deception? Science Digest 111:66–67, 1982

Trovillo PV: A history of lie detection. American Journal of Police Science 29:848–881, 1939

Trovillo PV: A history of lie detection (concluded from the previous issue). American Journal of Police Science 30:104–119, 1940

Twain M: On the decay of the art of lying (1896), in The Complete Works of Mark Twain. New York, Harper, 1923, pp 360–368

Underwood J: Truth, lies and resumes. The Birmingham News, August 22, 1993, pp D1, D10

Usher JA, Neisser V: Childhood amnesia and the beginnings of memory for your early life events. J Exp Psychol Gen 122:155–165, 1993

Vaillant GE: Theoretical hierarchy of adaptive ego mechanisms. Arch Gen Psychiatry 24:107–118, 1971

Vaillant GE, Vaillant CO: Natural history of male psychological health, XII: a 45-year study of predictors of successful aging at age 65. Am J Psychiatry 147:31–37, 1990

Vaillant GE, Bond M, Vaillant CO: An empirically validated hierarchy of defense mechanisms. Arch Gen Psychiatry 43:786–794, 1986

Vangelisti AL: Family secrets: forms, functions and correlates. Journal of Social and Personal Relationships 11:113–135, 1994

Vasek ME: Lying as a skill: the development of deception in children, in Deception: Perspectives on Human and Nonhuman Deceit. Edited by Mitchell RW, Thompson NS. Albany, NY, State University of New York Press, 1986, pp 271–292

Victor M, Adams RD, Collins GH: The Wernicke-Korsakoff Syndrome. Philadelphia, PA, FA Davis, 1971

Viederman M: Rene Magritte: coping with loss—reality and illusion. J Am Psychoanal Assoc 35:967–987, 1987

von Maur K, Warson KR, DeFord JW, et al: Munchausen's syndrome: a 30-year history of peregrination par excellence. South Med J 66:629–632, 1973

Vrij A: Credibility judgements of detectives: the impact of nonverbal behavior, social skills, and physical characteristics on impression formation. J Soc Psychol 133:601–610, 1993

Wakefield H, Underwager R: Recovered memories of alleged sexual abuse: lawsuits against parents. Behavioral Science and the Law 10:483–507, 1992

Wallerstein R: Observations on the personal myth and on theoretical perspectives in psychoanalysis, in The Personal Myth in Psychoanalytic Theory. Edited by Hartocollis P, Graham ID. Madison, CT, International Universities Press, 1991, pp 357–372

Warick LH, Warick ER: Transitional process and creativity in the life and art of Edvard Munch. J Am Acad Psychoanal 12:413–424, 1984

Warner F: What happened to the truth? Adweek's Marketing Week, October 28, 1991, pp 3–4

Webster H: Family Secrets: How Telling and Not Telling Affect Our Children, Our Relationships and Our Lives. Menlo Park, CA, Addison-Wesley, 1991

Webster's Seventh New Collegiate Dictionary. Springfield, MA, G & C Merriam Co, 1971

Weinberger DA, Schwartz GE, Davidson RJ: Low-anxious, high-anxious, and repressive coping styles: psychometric patterns and behavioral and psychological responses to stress. J Abnorm Psychol 88:369–380, 1979

Weingarten K: On lies, secrets, and not telling the truth: a training curriculum, in Secrets in Families and Family Therapy. Edited by Imber-Black E. New York, WW Norton, 1993, pp 373–389

Weinshel EM: Some observations on not telling the truth. J Am Psychoanal Assoc 27:503–531, 1979

Weinstein EA: Linguistic aspects of amnesia and confabulation. J Psychiatr Res 8:439–444, 1971

Wells CE: The hysterical personality and the feminine character: a study of Scarlett O'Hara. Compr Psychiatry 17:353–359, 1976

Wijsenbeek H, Nitzan I: The case of Peter, an impostor. Psychiatria Neurologia Neurochirurgia 71:193–202, 1968

Wilde O: The decay of lying: an observation (1892), in The Writings of Oscar Wilde: Intentions (Uniform Edition, Vol 6). New York, Keller, 1907, pp 5–63

Wile I: Lying as a biological and social phenomenon. Nervous Child 1:293–313, 1942

Williams M: Successful celebrities urge students to greatness. The Sunday Tennessean (Nashville), July 3, 1988, pp 1A–2A

Wimmer H, Gruber S, Perner J: Young children's conception of lying: moral intuition and denotation and connotation of "to lie." Developmental Psychology 21(6):993–995, 1985

Winnicott DW: CG Jung: Memories, Dreams, Reflections (book review). Int J Psychoanal 34:450–455, 1964

Witkin G: The hunt for a better lie detector: new technology probes the criminal mind. U.S. News and World Report 114(18):49, 1993

Wolf ES: The personal myth and the history of the self, in The Personal Myth in Psychoanalytic Theory. Edited by Hartocollis P, Graham ID. Madison, CT, International Universities Press, 1991, pp 89–107

Woolf M: The child's moral development, in Searchlights on Delinquency: New Psychoanalytic Studies. Edited by Eissler KR, Federn P. New York, International Universities Press, 1949, pp 263–272

Wright R: The Moral Animal: Evolutionary Psychology and Everyday Life. New York, Pantheon, 1994a

Wright R: Feminists, meet Mr. Darwin. New Republic 211(22):34–46, 1994b

Wyckham RC: Implied superiority claims. Journal of Advertising Research 27:54–63, 1987

Yapko MD: Suggestibility and repressed memories of abuse: a survey of psychotherapists' beliefs. Am J Clin Hypn 36:163–171, 1994

Yassa R: Munchausen's syndrome: a successfully treated case. Psychosomatics 19:242–243, 1978

Yorker BC: Nurses accused of murder. Am J Nurs 88:1327–1332, 1988

Ziv A: Children's behavior problems as viewed by teachers, psychologists, and children. Child Dev 41:871–879, 1970

Zuckerman M, Driver RE: Telling lies: verbal and nonverbal correlates of deception, in Multichannel Integrations of Nonverbal Behavior. Edited by Siegman AW, Feldstein S. Hillsdale, NJ, Erlbaum, 1984, pp 129–149

Zuckerman M, Koestner R, Alton AD: Learning to detect deception. J Pers Soc Psychol 46:519–528, 1984

Zuckerman M, Koestner R, Colella MJ: Learning to detect deception from three communication channels. Journal of Nonverbal Behavior 9:188–194, 1985

Index

Guilt, pseudologia fantastica
    and, 137
Guilty knowledge test (GKT),
    polygraph, 228–229

Habitual liars, 137–140,
    238–241. *See also*
    Compulsive lying
Halleck, Seymour, 114
Hamlyn, D. W., 38
Hand movements, 204
Hart, Gary, 11
Harvard University, 16
Hayano, David, 215–216
History, truth and deception
    in, 282
Histrionic personality
    disorder, 34, 110–116, 130
Hitler, Adolf, 258, 278
Hollender, Dr. Marc, 114
Homelessness, Munchausen
    behavior and, 164
Hoppe, Klaus, 57–58
Hulbert, Mark, 8
Human immunodeficiency
    virus (HIV), 14, 266
Humor
    as ego-defense mechanism,
        43
    humorous lies as
        classification of lying,
        29–30
    practical jokes as form of
        deceit, 92
Hydromorphine, 145
Hypochondriasis, as
    ego-defense mechanism,
    40

Hysteria. *See* Histrionic
    personality disorder

Identity
    creation of as motive for
        lying, 100–101
    impostors and, 153, 154–155
Idiosyncratic error, 200
Illustrators, body movements
    and deception, 203–204
Imposture
    characteristics of, 20–21
    childhood trauma and, 84
    con artists and, 158
    psychiatric studies of,
        148–155
    and sense of identity, 101
Impression management, 80–81
Impulse control
    borderline personality
        disorder and, 118–119
    pathological lying and,
        140–142, 274
    pharmacological treatment
        of, 245
    psychotherapy for lying
        and, 244
Incest. *See* Sexual abuse
Individuation
    and deceit in children,
        72–73, 275
    lying and process of, 20, 88
Information processing,
    unconscious and
    mechanism of, 36–37
Ingenuous, definition of, 26
Insight-oriented
    psychotherapy, 187